D1588329

C20449372

Video Atlas of
Intracranial Aneurysm Surgery

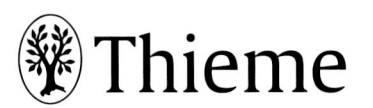

Video Atlas of Intracranial Aneurysm Surgery

Eric S. Nussbaum, MD
Chair, National Brain Aneurysm Center
St. Joseph's Hospital
St. Paul, Minnesota

Thieme
New York · Stuttgart

Thieme Medical Publishers, Inc.
333 Seventh Ave.
New York, NY 10001

Executive Editor: Kay Conerly
Managing Editor: Judith Tomat
Editorial Assistant: Leslie Feinberg
Editorial Director, Clinical Reference: Michael Wachinger
Production Editor: Kenneth L. Chumbley
International Production Director: Andreas Schabert
Senior Vice President, International Marketing and Sales: Cornelia Schulze
Vice President, Finance and Accounts: Sarah Vanderbilt
President: Brian D. Scanlan
Compositor: Prairie Papers Inc.
Printer: Everbest Printing Company

Medical Illustrator: Jennifer Pryll

Library of Congress Cataloging-in-Publication Data
Nussbaum, Eric S.
Video atlas of intracranial aneurysm surgery / Eric S. Nussbaum.
    p. ; cm.
  ISBN 978-1-60406-738-5 (alk. paper)–ISBN 978-1-60406-739-2 (e-ISBN)
  I. Title.
  [DNLM: 1. Intracranial Aneurysm—surgery—Atlases. 2. Microsurgery—Atlases. WL 17]

616.1′3300223—dc23

2012012801

Copyright © 2013 by Thieme Medical Publishers, Inc. This book, including all parts thereof, is legally protected by copyright. Any use, exploitation, or commercialization outside the narrow limits set by copyright legislation without the publisher's consent is illegal and liable to prosecution. This applies in particular to photostat reproduction, copying, mimeographing or duplication of any kind, translating, preparation of microfilms, and electronic data processing and storage.

Important note: Medical knowledge is ever-changing. As new research and clinical experience broaden our knowledge, changes in treatment and drug therapy may be required. The authors and editors of the material herein have consulted sources believed to be reliable in their efforts to provide information that is complete and in accord with the standards accepted at the time of publication. However, in view of the possibility of human error by the authors, editors, or publisher of the work herein or changes in medical knowledge, neither the authors, editors, nor publisher, nor any other party who has been involved in the preparation of this work, warrants that the information contained herein is in every respect accurate or complete, and they are not responsible for any errors or omissions or for the results obtained from use of such information. Readers are encouraged to confirm the information contained herein with other sources. For example, readers are advised to check the product information sheet included in the package of each drug they plan to administer to be certain that the information contained in this publication is accurate and that changes have not been made in the recommended dose or in the contraindications for administration. This recommendation is of particular importance in connection with new or infrequently used drugs.

Some of the product names, patents, and registered designs referred to in this book are in fact registered trademarks or proprietary names even though specific reference to this fact is not always made in the text. Therefore, the appearance of a name without designation as proprietary is not to be construed as a representation by the publisher that it is in the public domain.

Printed in China

5 4 3 2 1

ISBN 978-1-60406-738-5
eISBN 978-1-60406-739-2

For my wife, Leslie, and our children, Toby, Poppy, Frank, Heather, and Bailey.

Corporate Acknowledgments

The author and publisher thank the following organizations for their kind support of this publication:

Leica Microsystems
Heerbrugg, Switzerland

The National Brain Aneurysm Center
Saint Joseph's Hospital
St. Paul, Minnesota, USA

Contents

C20449372

Video Contents

1 Surgical Approaches to Intracranial Aneurysms

No video

2 Aneurysms of the Anterior Cerebral Artery

VIDEO 1

Small, unruptured, anteriorly-directed ACOMMA aneurysm approached via a left-sided pterional craniotomy. The patient had previously undergone clipping of a right middle cerebral artery aneurysm and a ruptured basilar apex aneurysm from a right-sided approach.

VIDEO 2

Unruptured, superiorly-directed ACOMMA aneurysm tucked up in anterior interhemispheric fissure treated via a left-sided approach. The video demonstrates exposure of the optic apparatus, opening of the proximal Sylvian fissure, and opening of the anterior interhemispheric fissure to spare the gyrus rectus. After clipping, a small amount of gortex is used to reinforce the bulbous area remaining along the superior aspect of the reconstructed anterior communicating artery.

VIDEO 3

Small ACOMMA aneurysm treated from the left side following a recent subarachnoid hemorrhage. The aneurysm is directed ventrally and superiorly. A small amount of focal resection of the medial gyrus rectus is used to expose the aneurysm. An intra-operative angiogram is shown as well.

VIDEO 4

Complex, multilobulated ACOMMA aneurysm treated from the right side. The inferiorly and ventrally directed lobes are clipped independently, and the gyrus rectus is left intact. A mini-clip is used to obliterate a small amount of residual near-neck at the end.

VIDEO 5

This is an unedited version of the previous video which is included to show every aspect of the intradural portion of the operation including exposure, dissection, and clipping of the aneurysm. This is longer (approximately 20 minutes), unedited, and without narration.

VIDEO 6

A complex, wide-necked, ruptured ACOMMA aneurysm approached from the right side, despite the dominant A1 being on the left because the ACOMMA complex was rotated such that the aneurysm would have been more difficult to clip from the left. We begin by identifying both A1's. Temporary clips are used on both A1's to allow for dissection of the aneurysm neck.

VIDEO 7

Redo, recurrent ACOMMA aneurysm in a patient who had previously undergone bilateral craniotomies at another institution many years earlier following a subarachnoid hemorrhage for a ruptured ACOMMA aneurysm. There were two separate components to the recurrence, one directed inferiorly and a second larger lobule directed superiorly. Given the expected scarring from the prior hemorrhage and multiple craniotomies, a small subfrontal exposure was performed on the right side. The optic nerves are identified, and one of the old clips is demonstrated. The inferior lobule is white and easily exposed. The larger superior lobe is thin walled and exposed with a small amount of subpial resection. The lesions are clipped separately, sparing of the perforators is illustrated, and an intraoperative angiogram is included.

VIDEO 8

Small, ruptured, distal ACA aneurysm treated through an interhemispheric approach. At the start, a large bridging vein is encountered, necessitating slight forward extension of the craniotomy. The interhemispheric fissure is opened, and proximal control is achieved by dissecting past the aneurysm to reach the ACA. The inferior aspect of the falx is opened to widen the exposure. A small amount of clot is left on the aneurysm dome, and the callosomarginal branch is separated from the dome to allow for clipping of the aneurysm.

VIDEO 9

Distal ACA aneurysm exposed through an interhemispheric approach. The dome is adherent to the contralateral frontal lobe, and a small amount of subpial resection is used, leaving the dome undisturbed. As the clip closes, one can appreciate the callosomarginal artery coming into view. The clip blades are rotated to properly inspect the anatomy, and a second micro clip is used to obliterate a small residual near-neck remnant.

VIDEO 10

A ruptured, complex, bilobed distal ACA aneurysm treated with full mobilization of the aneurysm dome, leaving a small amount of clot on the dome. Multiple clips are used to reconstruct the aneurysm.

VIDEO 11

An unusual aneurysm of the A1 segment is exposed through a right-sided pterional craniotomy. Note the preservation of a subfrontal vein running along the exposure as well as careful dissection of the nearby perforators including Heubner. The aneurysm dome is freed from the underlying optic chiasm prior to clipping. Intraoperative angiography is included.

3 Paraclinoid Aneurysms

▶ VIDEO 12

A small, left-sided carotid ophthalmic aneurysm in a very young patient is exposed through a left pterional approach. The dura over the clinoid is reflected to create a small flap over the optic nerve. The ultrasonic bone-cutting device is utilized to thin the clinoid. The falciform ligament is opened, and the optic nerve is mobilized to visualize and dissect the aneurysm neck and the ophthalmic artery origin. ICG video angiography is performed at the end.

▶ VIDEO 13

Small carotid ophthalmic aneurysm in a case of suspected subarachnoid hemorrhage. The anterior clinoid is removed, the falciform ligament is opened, and a robust view of the aneurysm is provided. Formal intraoperative angiography is included.

▶ VIDEO 14

Posterior paraclinoid aneurysm causing partial 3rd nerve palsy. After the anterior clinoid process has been removed, a right-angled, fenestrated clip is used, placing the internal carotid artery in the fenestration to reconstruct the artery. Care is taken to keep the clip blades well below the origins of the posterior communicating and anterior choroidal arteries.

▶ VIDEO 15

A large paraclinoid aneurysm compressing the optic nerve is treated through a right-sided pterional craniotomy. The aneurysm is dissected from the optic apparatus. Note the sharp dissection to free the A1 segment of the anterior cerebral artery from the aneurysm to allow for proper clipping. The aneurysm is clipped, and then the blood within the aneurysm is aspirated to decompress the optic nerve.

4 Supraclinoid Internal Carotid Artery Aneurysms

▶ VIDEO 16

Right-sided pterional approach for posterior communicating artery aneurysm. The internal carotid artery is yellow-white and atheromatous in comparison to the thin-walled, red aneurysm. Sharp dissection is used to free the anterior choroidal artery from the aneurysm neck, and the dome of the aneurysm is fully mobilized. The fetal-type posterior communicating artery is carefully separated prior to aneurysm clipping.

VIDEO 17

This is an interesting case of multiple aneurysms. There is a large, left-sided posterior communicating artery aneurysm and a smaller, thin-walled anterior choroidal aneurysm with the choroidal artery "sandwiched" between them. The larger aneurysm is dissected and clipped with a fenestrated clip that places the anterior choroidal artery itself, as well as the associated small aneurysm, in the fenestration. Once applied, the larger aneurysm is collapsed and the vascular anatomy can be more thoroughly inspected. This allows for further deep dissection and then replacement of the clip at a better angle. A second clip is similarly applied that allows for further, deep dissection, and then the clip can be reapplied more carefully and precisely. Finally, the choroidal aneurysm is treated. Note the superior cerebellar artery that is well seen in the deep background.

VIDEO 18

A large, left-sided, posterior communicating artery aneurysm is exposed through a pterional approach. The neck is dissected. When the internal carotid artery is retracted medially, the basilar artery is well-visualized. Because the patient presented with a 3rd nerve palsy, the aneurysm is aspirated and then coagulated down to facilitate recovery of the compressive cranial neuropathy. After clipping of the posterior communicating artery aneurysm, a small, broad-based anterior choroidal artery aneurysm at the origin of a duplicated choroidal artery is dissected and clipped with a tiny AVM clip.

VIDEO 19

A small, unruptured, anterior choroidal artery aneurysm is exposed on the right side through a pterional craniotomy. The video demonstrates sharp dissection to open the proximal Sylvian fissure. The aneurysm is aggressively mobilized, and an accessory choroidal artery is meticulously dissected from the aneurysm neck to allow for clip placement. Note the time and effort taken to dissect the vessel from the aneurysm and then to ensure it has not been kinked or injured by the clip. Also of note is that the lateral retraction of the carotid is utilized to properly visualize the posterior communicating artery with all its branches.

VIDEO 20

This patient has numerous small aneurysms. A right-sided pterional craniotomy is performed. Aneurysms of the anterior temporal artery, posterior communicating artery, and anterior choroidal artery are readily exposed. The small choroidal aneurysm is nestled between a good-sized choroidal artery and a smaller, secondary choroidal vessel. Its dissection is complicated by the anatomy of the M1 segment hiding it to some degree and the angle of the internal carotid artery itself. Meticulous dissection is used to fully expose and clip the choroidal aneurysm. Finally, a sessile basilar apex aneurysm is wrapped with gortex, and a contralateral superior cerebellar aneurysm is explored. A decision is made to leave the SCA lesion to be treated at the time of a contralateral craniotomy that was planned to address multiple left-sided aneurysms.

5 Aneurysms of the Carotid Bifurcation

6 Aneurysms of the Middle Cerebral Artery

exposed by opening the interhemispheric fissure. Sharp dissection right along the dome is used to free the aneurysm in preparation for clip reconstruction.

⟳ VIDEO 36)

An unusual peripheral MCA aneurysm in a patient presenting with speech difficulty due to TIAs. The aneurysm is fully exposed, revealing an en passage MCA branch running below it and clearly separate inflow and outflow to the aneurysm. Attempted clipping repeatedly compromised the outflow on intraoperative angiography. The superficial temporal artery was therefore anastomosed to the efferent branch immediately distal to the aneurysm. The aneurysm is then trapped, opened, and excised completely.

7 Aneurysms of the Basilar Artery

⟳ VIDEO 37)

Ruptured small basilar apex aneurysm treated through right-sided pterional approach. Working between the 3rd nerve and internal carotid artery, the basilar apex is exposed. Note how the white basilar artery transitions to the very thin-walled, red aneurysm neck. The suction is used to retract the carotid, providing exposure to the upper basilar artery. The neck is dissected carefully, and a large perforator running along the aneurysm is protected. A bayoneted clip is used to treat the aneurysm. A final overview shows the Sylvian opening and the extent of the exposure of the frontal and temporal lobes.

⟳ VIDEO 38)

Larger basilar apex aneurysm exposed through a predominantly subtemporal approach. The tentorium is cut and tacked back with a suture. The P1 and its perforators are nicely visualized. Dissection proceeds behind the aneurysm, dissecting free the perforators from the back wall of the aneurysm. A fenestrated clip is applied with the P1 in the fenestration. A small amount of residual far neck is identified, but we use the opportunity to free perforators from the far neck. The clip is opened and advanced, and then a second clip is applied above the P1 for completion. Note the meticulous dissection of all thalamoperforating vessels behind the aneurysm and along the ipsilateral P1. After clipping, note how the clip blades are gently rotated to allow for clear visualization of the perforators to ensure none has been caught in the clip blades.

⟳ VIDEO 39)

Wide-necked basilar apex aneurysm exposed through half-half approach and clipped from a more subtemporal view. The Sylvian fissure is widely opened, developing gradually the corridors between the carotid and 3rd nerve and between the carotid and optic nerve. The M1 segment is dissected from the temporal lobe to mobilize the temporal lobe. The aneurysm is inspected from a ventral perspective, and a decision is made to elevate the temporal lobe to add a subtemporal exposure to properly view the back wall of the aneurysm. The tentorium is cut and sutured back. The perforators are then dissected from the back wall of the aneurysm after a temporary clip has been placed on the upper basilar artery. The aneurysm is treated with a fenestrated clip, placing the P1 in the fenestration. A small amount of near neck is left open in the fenestration along with the P1, and this is treated with a second short clip applied above the P1.

▶ VIDEO 40

A partially thrombosed, thrombotic aneurysm of the SCA is treated in a patient presenting with a 3rd nerve palsy. A subtemporal approach is utilized. The aneurysm is visible as a dark, rounded mass with the 3rd nerve stretched over and adherent to the dome. A fenestrated clip is used, placing the 3rd nerve in the fenestration to reconstruct the lateral aspect of the basilar artery and occlude the aneurysm.

▶ VIDEO 41

A small superior cerebellar artery aneurysm is exposed through a left-sided pterional approach. The aneurysm is dissected by working between the internal carotid artery and the 3rd cranial nerve. Because of the limited working room through this corridor, the aneurysm is clipped by bringing a clip down through the optico-carotid triangle, while watching though the space between the internal carotid artery and the 3rd nerve as the clip blades close the aneurysm. A final overview of the amount of the pterional exposure is provided as well.

▶ VIDEO 42

Rare case of a sidewall dissecting aneurysm of the basilar artery treated through a combined presigmoid-subtemporal approach. After ligation of the superior petrosal sinus, the tentorium is divided completely to expose the 4th nerve. Note retractors on cerebellum and undersurface of temporal lobe. The arachnoid is opened between the 5th nerve and the 7–8 nerve complex to expose the proximal basilar trunk. Note the gradual development of working corridors above and below the 5th nerve. The aneurysm is seen and dissected above the 5th nerve and deep to cranial nerve IV. A large basilar artery perforator is freed from the back wall of the aneurysm, and two clips are applied parallel to the long axis of the basilar artery to obliterate the aneurysm.

8 Posterior Inferior Cerebellar Artery Aneurysms

▶ VIDEO 43

Far lateral suboccipital approach is utilized to expose a small PICA aneurysm. Note the lower cranial nerve rootlets and the small PICA itself running along the aneurysm dome. A fenestrated clip is utilized, placing the PICA itself in the fenestration. Note the excellent exposure with only minimal cerebellar retraction.

9 Special Considerations: Giant Aneurysms, Bypasses, Previously Coiled Lesions, and Rare Locations

Giant Aneurysms and Bypasses

exposed, and with a temporary clip on the supraclinoid ICA distal to the aneurysm but proximal to the PCOMM artery, suction decompression is used to soften the aneurysm, which is then obliterated with several long clips stacked above its atheromatous neck.

▶ VIDEO 49

This video demonstrates the use of a radial artery graft from the cervical external carotid artery to the MCA to treat a giant, calcified, MCA bifurcation aneurysm. The distal anastomosis is shown using a running suture technique. Note the delicate handling of the MCA branch. Once the anastomosis is completed, a temporary clip is applied to the distal M1 segment, and intraoperative angiography is performed to confirm filling of the MCA branches from the bypass. This is then replaced with a permanent clip to treat the aneurysm.

▶ VIDEO 50

Giant, peripheral, thrombotic MCA aneurysm causing significant mass effect on dominant hemisphere. The peripheral Sylvian fissure is opened to reveal the giant aneurysm as a bluish-green mass. The inflow and outflow vessels are isolated, and the STA is then anastomosed to the outflow MCA branch. After intraoperative angiography confirms patency of the bypass, the aneurysm is trapped and cut open. The ultrasonic aspirator is used to remove a large amount of thrombus from the aneurysm, nicely decompressing the brain.

▶ VIDEO 51

Giant, calcified, atheromatous aneurysm involving the distal M1 segment is exposed though a pterional craniotomy. A large STA is anastomosed to one of the M2 branches just beyond the MCA bifurcation. This is performed with 10-0 suture as shown. At this point, the M1 segment is occluded just proximal to the aneurysm, and a Drake tourniquet is applied to the distal M1 segment just beyond the aneurysm neck and proximal to the MCA bifurcation. This was left in place to trap the aneurysm the next day, but postoperative angiography demonstrated complete thrombosis of the aneurysm. Simple proximal occlusion was utilized, and the tourniquet was removed.

▶ VIDEO 52

This video demonstrates the use of an STA-MCA bypass to augment flow in preparation for occlusion of the internal carotid artery in a young patient who presents with a severe subarachnoid hemorrhage from a dissecting pseudoaneurysm involving the entire length of the supraclinoid carotid artery. The STA is dissected, and then the craniotomy is shown with the STA in its natural position overlying the opening. The dura is opened, and a cortical MCA branch is exposed and isolated. The STA is prepared, and the MCA branch is temporarily occluded and then opened. The anastomosis is performed using interrupted 10-0 suture. At this point, the supraclinoid ICA is occluded at the level of the optic nerve proximal to the aneurysm. Intraoperative angiography shows filling of the ipsilateral MCA territory via the bypass. There is limited residual filling of the ICA through the PCOMM artery on vertebral angiography. The opposite ICA fills both anterior cerebral arteries with minimal contribution to the ipsilateral MCA territory.

Previously Coiled Aneurysms

⟳ VIDEO 53

A large, previously ruptured, previously coiled MCA aneurysm is exposed by a sharp opening of the Sylvian fissure after the STA has been dissected out (in the event a bypass should be necessary). Note the scarring in the fissure from the old hemorrhage and the preservation of the Sylvian veins. The proximal fissure is opened for control, and an incidental ICA bifurcation aneurysm is dissected and clipped. The large aneurysm is then explored, and coils are noted coming down toward the aneurysm neck. Multiple clips are used to close the neck, with a single coil being "trapped" in the largest clip. Intraoperative angiography reveals some residual filling, so an additional clip is applied. A final angiogram shows complete occlusion of the aneurysm.

⟳ VIDEO 54

This patient suffered a severe SAH with a temporal lobe hematoma from a MCA aneurysm. The aneurysm was coiled at another institution, and the patient was transferred when he suffered neurological deterioration due to edema around the hematoma. A decision was made to take the patient to the operating room for evacuation of the hematoma. A lateral Sylvian opening is shown coming down on the aneurysm at the MCA bifurcation. Although the dome is secured with coils, residual filling of the aneurysm neck and up along the back wall is identified. The aneurysm is obliterated with two clips below the coil mass. Intraoperative angiography shows complete exclusion of the aneurysm.

⟳ VIDEO 55

This patient suffered a severe SAH from a distal ACA aneurysm that was coiled and then recoiled a year later when it recurred. When the aneurysm recurred, the patient was referred for surgical therapy, which is shown through an interhemispheric fissure approach. Note the coils sitting free in the subarachnoid space outside the aneurysm dome. The neck is exposed, and the pericallosal and callosomarginal arteries are isolated. A clip is worked across the neck, below the coil mass, to obliterate the aneurysm.

Rare Locations

⟳ VIDEO 56

This is a very unusual case of a large, lenticulostriate aneurysm that ruptured causing an intracerebral and intraventricular hemorrhage in a young patient with moya moya. She was seen at another institution where an ec-ic bypass was attempted but was unsuccessful. A decision was made to attempt to clip the aneurysm and to perform a new bypass to decrease future risk of ischemic or hemorrhagic complication. First, a small cortical opening is made in the inferior temporal gyrus, and dissection is carried down toward the aneurysm. Intraoperative angiography is performed with a clip in place as a marker to guide the dissection. Before reaching the aneurysm, the Sylvian fissure is opened sharply to provide access to the M1 segment and the moya moya vessels, to achieve some degree of proximal control. At this point, the aneurysm dome and neck are dissected, and the aneurysm is treated with primary neck clipping. Intraoperative angiography is repeated. Finally, the frontal branch of the STA is dissected (the parietal branch having been sacrificed during the prior attempted bypass), and an STA-MCA anastomosis is performed using 10-0 interrupted suture, as illustrated.

VIDEO 57

A rare, ruptured aneurysm of a posterolateral cervical spinal artery is exposed through a cervical laminoplasty. The dura is opened to reveal a thick, subarachnoid clot. Hematoma is removed and an abnormal, small, corkscrew vessel is identified proximal and distal to the aneurysm. The lesion is trapped with SSEP and MEP monitoring. The true aneurysm is then dissected, excised, and opened.

10 General Principles of Aneurysm Surgery: Nuances and Advice for Successful Outcomes and Complication Avoidance

No video

Preface

Neurosurgeons have always been fascinated by the management of intracranial aneurysms (IAs) because of the elegant and technically demanding nature of their surgical repair. Most neurovascular surgeons would agree that the ideal treatment for an IA remains surgical neck clipping, assuming that the surgery can be performed without complication. Unfortunately, a number of factors have combined to challenge the aneurysm surgeon's ability to achieve reliably good results.

With the progressive refinement of endovascular techniques, the introduction of newer devices (including stents, remodeling balloons, and coated coils), and with the early results of the ISAT study suggesting that patients with ruptured IAs fared better with endovascular treatment, a growing percentage of IAs are now being treated endovascularly. At the same time, the results of the International Study of Unruptured Intracranial Aneurysms trial suggested that unruptured aneurysms may carry a more benign natural history than had been previously appreciated, tempering enthusiasm for recommending treatment to patients with smaller, incidentally discovered lesions. Together, these issues have decreased significantly the number of IAs undergoing open microsurgical clipping.

As the amount of open aneurysm surgery has decreased, technical facility and comfort levels with these procedures have similarly declined. And as a result, younger neurosurgeons and neurosurgical residents are being exposed to a progressively decreasing volume of aneurysm surgery. Without doubt, this decreasing volume will, over time, continue to erode proficiency with the fine microsurgical techniques required to treat IAs. In many programs, the average chief resident may go through an entire year without participating in the clipping of a complex posterior circulation lesion or a giant aneurysm. More disconcerting, however, is the limited volume of routine aneurysm surgery to which trainees are being exposed.

In response to a perceived need for greater exposure to the microsurgical techniques necessary to treat IAs, I have assembled a collection of carefully chosen operative images and videos that cover the spectrum of IA surgery. Lesions of varying sizes, complexities, and locations are included, but an emphasis has been placed on the types of aneurysms that might be encountered on a routine basis by neurosurgeons treating IAs. In the accompanying text, focused discussion and tables highlight the critical elements associated with treating the aneurysms shown in the photos and videos.

In my opinion, too much time is spent at meetings and in the literature addressing the treatment of the most complicated and challenging aneurysms. For the reader interested in a book that focuses on these complex cases, there are other good works that represent a testament to the outstanding technical skills of their authors. This book is very different, highlighting the treatment of routine IAs and the techniques that have allowed us to achieve good results on a regular basis at our center.

Over the past decade and a half, I have had the opportunity to evaluate more than 10,000 IAs, selecting roughly one-fifth of these for microsurgical repair. This has provided a unique opportunity to develop and refine a variety of intraoperative techniques and strategies that have produced reliably successful outcomes in the majority of cases. Based on this experience, the current work offers a personal perspective of my preferred surgical methods for treating IAs. Yet, no matter how well-written and well-illustrated, no standard text can fully capture the art and spirit of a surgical procedure. The addition of surgical video represents an invaluable tool for expanding the educational process by demonstrating the microsurgical anatomy in a way that cannot be captured by text and still images alone. Nevertheless, working directly in the operating room with an experienced vascular neurosurgeon will always remain an irreplaceable portion of the training of dedicated aneurysm surgeons in the future.

Today, with our better understanding of the relatively benign natural history of many unruptured lesions, and with the continually expanding role of endovascular therapy, the aneurysm surgeon must produce far better results than did his/her predecessors to justify treating IAs through open microsurgery. Such results can only be achieved through judicious patient selection, meticulous intraoperative technique, and excellent postoperative care. It is hoped that this work will be of value to those younger surgeons who accept this challenge.

Acknowledgments

I wish that Dr. Charles Drake could have seen this atlas. I hope that he would have enjoyed it. I know he would have called me to say it would have worked better for the basilar tip aneurysm in Video 38 if I'd chosen an 8mm clip and filed down the tips "just a touch." It's impossible to describe how much I learned just sitting in his office, talking about complex aneurysm surgery, and reviewing old angiograms from his files. It's a debt I can never repay.

I would like to give special thanks to Mike Madison, Jim Goddard, and Jeff Lassig for their expert endovascular assistance and for all the intraoperative angiograms!

I could not do my job without the unparalleled assistance of Jody Lowary, who consistently demonstrates an incredible dedication to our patients, and Tariq Janjua, one of the finest neurointensivists in the world.

I owe so much to my amazing wife (a distinguished neurosurgeon in her own right) and children who graciously tolerate the long hours and still provide me with their overwhelming support.

Finally, thanks to Kay Conerly with Thieme for keeping things on track.

1 Surgical Approaches to Intracranial Aneurysms

There are a limited number of standard surgical approaches that enable the neurovascular surgeon to treat almost all intracranial aneurysms. These approaches represent the basis for exposing even the most complex of aneurysms, and the aneurysm surgeon should become facile with their performance. Under most circumstances, the experienced surgeon can complete these exposures in under one-half hour.

▪ Pterional

The pterional approach is one of the most versatile exposures available to the neurosurgeon. When performed properly, this approach affords the surgeon access to all aneurysms of the anterior circulation (with the exception of distal anterior and distal middle cerebral lesions) as well as most aneurysms involving the upper basilar artery. The approach also provides access to lesions involving the anterior and middle cranial fossae, including those of the cribriform plate, suprasellar cistern, and interpeduncular region.

As a general rule, the head is secured in a radiolucent frame to allow for intraoperative angiography. The malar eminence is positioned superiorly, and the head is extended slightly and rotated 30 to 45 degrees from the vertical axis depending on the exact location and orientation of the aneurysm being treated. Some of the nuances regarding positioning for particular aneurysm locations will be discussed individually in the ensuing chapters.

Several skin incisions can be utilized, although we have preferred an incision that begins in front of the ear at the level of the zygoma and stays behind the hairline, curving gently up to the midline. The temporalis fascia and muscle are divided sharply and reflected forward to expose the pterion, the orbital rim, and the frontal process of the zygoma (**Fig. 1.1A**). A cuff of fascia can be left attached to the skull to allow for resuspension of the temporalis muscle at the conclusion of the procedure.

Several burr holes are placed strategically to facilitate raising the bone flap. The exact number and location are a matter of the surgeon's preference, although we find it helpful if one hole is placed at the "keyhole," and as a rule, we prefer three holes, as illustrated in **Fig. 1.1A**.

A small bone flap, providing exposure of the frontal and temporal lobes and centered on the Sylvian fissure, suffices in most cases. Since the work in aneurysm surgery is generally being performed under the brain or through a fissure, we have avoided overly large flaps that add little to visualization and place additional exposed brain at risk for inadvertent injury. One exception is in the setting of severe subarachnoid hemorrhage (SAH), when a larger flap may be necessary for decompressive purposes and to avoid an overly swollen brain from herniating out through a small opening, obscuring visualization and precluding a safe operation.

One of the most critical aspects of the procedure is the adequate drilling of the skull base to provide a low, flat exposure without excessive brain retraction (**Fig. 1.1B**). The dura should be elevated from the lateral sphenoid wing, the orbital rim, and orbital roof. We use retractors to protect the frontal and temporal dura while aggressively drilling the lateral sphenoid wing as well as the orbital bone. At this point, the dura can be elevated from the deeper aspect of the sphenoid wing, and the medial sphenoid wing as well as a portion of the anterior clinoid process can be removed as needed. A combination of bone wax and topical hemostatic agents may be required to achieve hemostasis prior to dural opening. Of note, the surgeon should be careful to remove the prominent ridges along the orbital roof, particularly when accessing deeper, midline aneurysms, such as those of the anterior communicating and basilar arteries. Often, we end up exposing the periorbita while thinning down the orbital roof. In these instances, the periorbita should be left intact if possible. At times, the orbital fat is encountered, and we have not had any ocular complications in such cases, although the eye does tend to become more swollen in the early postoperative period.

The dura is opened in a curvilinear fashion based on the Sylvian fissure and tented up with sutures. The degrees of frontal and temporal exposure are tailored to the individual aneurysm being treated. For anterior communicating and paraclinoid lesions, a greater degree of frontal exposure is needed. For middle cerebral aneurysms, a more even exposure of the frontal and temporal lobes is appropriate.

At this point, we generally bring in the operating microscope. We have never favored using loupes in opening the Sylvian fissure or in elevating the frontal lobe, as the magnification and illumination of the microscope provide a superior alternative. The lateral aspect of the Sylvian fissure is opened to release cerebrospinal fluid (CSF) and begin the dissection (**Fig. 1.1C**). We generally use a microknife to open the arachnoid and then a pair of jeweler's forceps to begin the dissection. Sylvian veins are preserved whenever possible.

At this point, the exact aneurysm location being treated will determine the next steps. If the aneurysm arises at the middle cerebral bifurcation, the Sylvian opening is deepened and extended as needed to achieve proximal control and expose the aneurysm. When dealing with an anterior communicating, paraclinoid, or supraclinoid internal carotid artery (ICA) aneurysm, the frontal lobe can be gently elevated to expose the optico-carotid region. Arachnoid is sharply opened as illustrated in many of the included videos, and the surgeon should patiently allow CSF to drain, providing good brain relaxation in most cases (**Fig. 1.1D**).

The key to maximizing the safety and versatility of the pterional approach is the wide opening of all necessary arachnoid membranes at this point. Arachnoid bands tether the exposed structures, including the brain itself and associated arteries, veins, and cranial nerves. When retracting on the brain, the arachnoid transmits tension to any tethered structure, potentially risking injury. To avoid this risk, the surgeon should sharply divide the arachnoid to free the exposed structures and limit the transmitted tension. First, the arachnoid over the optic nerve and ICA should be taken down. The

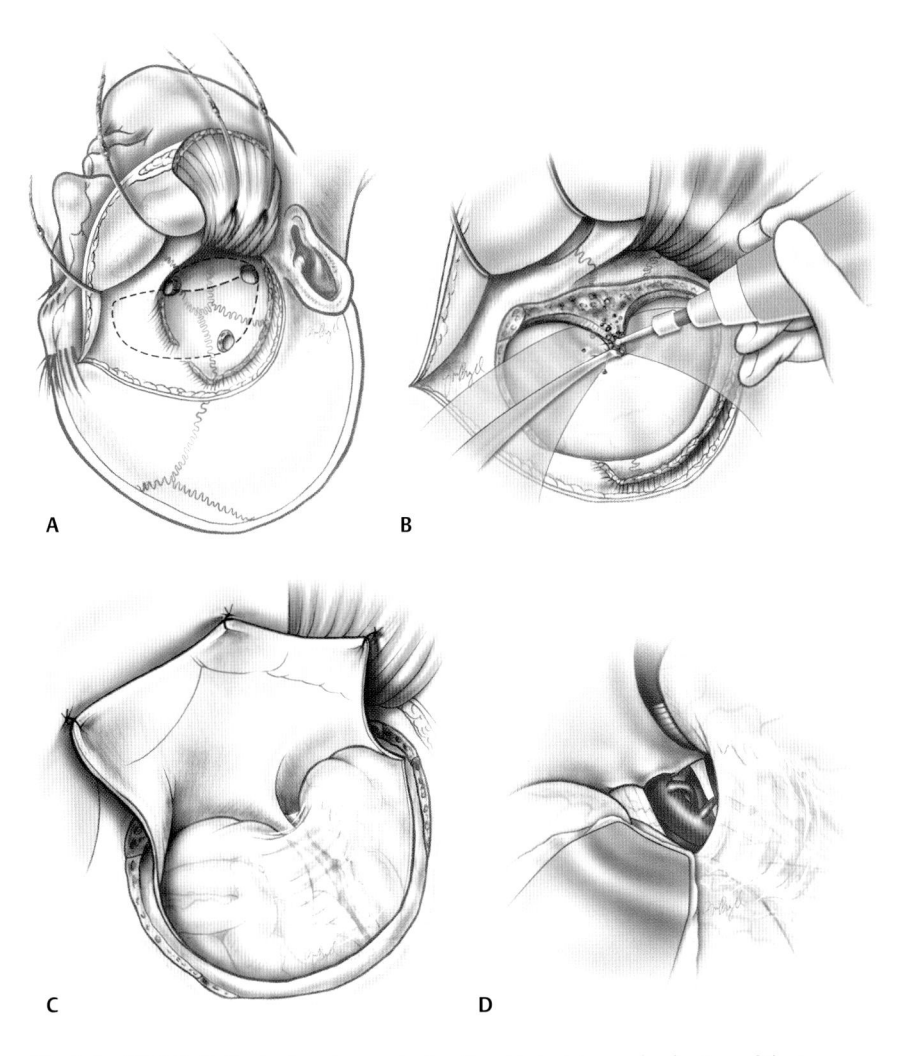

Fig. 1.1 **(A)** Artist's illustration demonstrating the skin incision and reflection of the temporalis muscle and fascia to reveal the underlying skull. The extent of the craniotomy is shown in orange. Additional bone is then drilled to provide a lower exposure, as shown in green. **(B)** The dura has been elevated from the floor of the anterior cranial fossa and sphenoid wing. A high-speed drill is used to remove the sphenoid wing while retractors protect the frontal and temporal dura. **(C)** The dura has been opened in curvilinear fashion based on the Sylvian fissure and tented up with suture. The frontal and temporal lobes are revealed and the Sylvian fissure exposed. **(D)** With the medial aspect of the Sylvian fissure opened, the supraclinoid ICA and optic nerve are visualized through the operating microscope.

proximal Sylvian fissure can be opened to whatever extent is needed to allow for exposure of the critical anatomy. For example, to treat a paraclinoid aneurysm, only the proximal fissure needs to be opened, whereas to reach a carotid bifurcation lesion, the fissure should be opened to expose at least the proximal M1 segment.

The optic nerve is freed of all attachments to the ipsilateral frontal lobe, being careful to protect the recurrent artery of Heubner, which may be crossing the field just deep to this point. The olfactory tract should be freed as needed to avoid injury to it. In its fullest expression, the pterional exposure affords a dramatic and wide view of numerous critical areas of the brain.

As will be described next, the use of several adjunctive measures can further widen the anatomy that can be reached through this versatile exposure.

▪ Orbitocranial and Orbitozygomatic

The orbitocranial and orbitozygomatic approaches are variations of the pterional approach that widen the anatomical exposure by incorporating additional removal of bony structures from the skull base (**Fig. 1.2**).

The orbitocranial (OC) approach adds removal of the orbital rim and orbital roof to the standard pterional approach as described above. The periorbita is exposed fully, and when the dura is opened, it is aggressively sutured down flat, depressing the periorbita and maximizing the exposure. We have found the OC approach to be helpful when treating highly positioned anterior communicating aneurysms, particularly those pointing superiorly and posteriorly. The lower angle of approach minimizes the need for deep brain retraction. In fact, after opening the dura, the surgeon can often immediately visualize the optic nerve and internal carotid artery with minimal or no brain retraction. When treating larger paraclinoid aneurysms, the OC approach brings the surgeon that much closer to the critical anatomy.

The orbitozygomatic (OZ) approach extends this concept one step further by taking down the zygoma as well as additional bone from the lateral orbital wall (**Fig. 1.2**). This additional exposure helps with deeper aneurysms, such as those involving the basilar apex. The exposure can be performed as a one-step maneuver, removing the pterional bone flap along with the orbital rim, orbital roof, and zygomatic process. In our practice, we have been more comfortable using a two-step approach. First, a standard pterional craniotomy is performed. Additional dissection of the zygomatic arch is added. Once the pterional flap has been raised, the dura is elevated from the orbital roof, which is then removed along with the orbital rim and the zygomatic process as a second bone piece. Each approach has its advocates; surgeons should become facile with their preferred technique. With experience, either option should add no more than 15 minutes to the standard pterional exposure. One concern with the OZ is the propensity for temporalis wasting that can be associated with the additional dissection. A careful subperiosteal approach and meticulous resuspension of the temporalis muscle will help to avoid this issue.

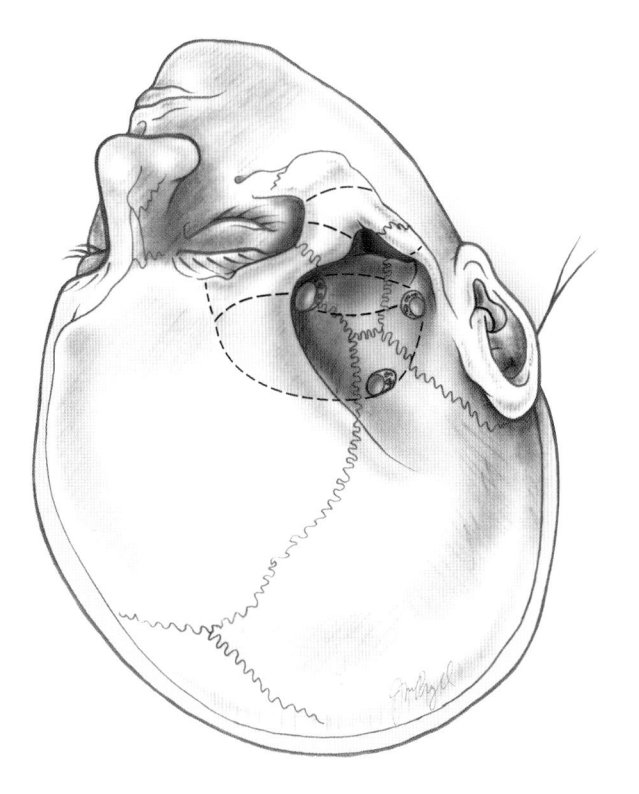

Fig. 1.2 Artist's drawing demonstrating the previously described pterional craniotomy (orange) with additional bone removal (green). The orbitocranial approach includes removal of the orbital rim and a portion of the frontal process of the zygoma (yellow) as well as the orbital roof. The orbitozygomatic approach further extends the bone removal to include the zygomatic bar, as shown in purple.

■ Parasagittal Interhemispheric

The parasagittal interhemispheric approach is utilized to treat distal anterior cerebral artery aneurysms. Although the exposure traditionally calls for a generous flap that spans the coronal suture, we have generally used a small flap on the right side that sits in front of this landmark. The use of frameless stereotactic guidance helps to direct the surgeon's flap and approach.

Several burr holes are placed along the midline (**Fig. 1.3A**). A parasagittal flap is raised, and the dura is opened based on the superior sagittal sinus, carefully preserving any bridging veins (**Fig. 1.3B**). Once the interhemispheric fissure has been accessed, the fissure is opened as needed under the operating microscope, coming down to reach the anterior cerebral artery branches. These can be followed to the aneurysm. More detail regarding this approach is provided in Chapter 2.

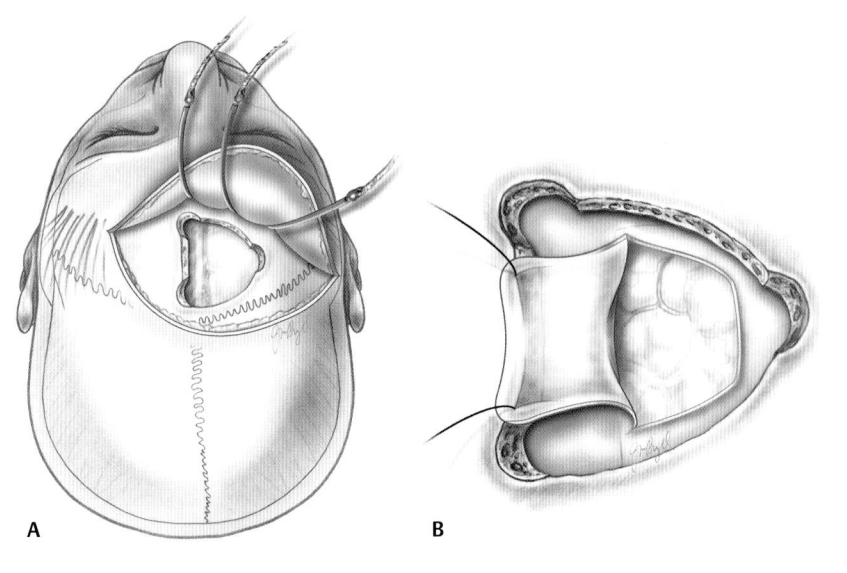

Fig. 1.3 **(A)** The anterior interhemispheric approach is illustrated showing the limited skin incision and small craniotomy that exposes the superior sagittal sinus. **(B)** The dura has been opened based on the sinus and reflected back to expose the underlying cortical surface and provide access to the interhemispheric fissure.

◾ Subtemporal

The subtemporal approach is most useful for aneurysms of the upper basilar artery. As perfected by Drake, the exposure can be performed through a short vertical incision beginning in front of the ear and extending to the superior temporal line, a so-called "tic" incision. The temporalis fascia and muscle are split, and a small craniotomy, coming right down to the middle fossa floor, is made. The dura is then opened flush with the middle fossa floor, and the temporal lobe is gently elevated with several retractors to distribute the retraction force over as large an area as possible. The use of CSF drainage is important, and patience is necessary as the temporal lobe is gradually elevated until the incisura is exposed.

At this point, the third nerve can be seen, and the arachnoid is opened, giving the surgeon a glimpse of the posterior cerebral artery (PCA) and lateral aspect of the brainstem. The tentorium is generally divided just behind the insertion of the fourth cranial nerve and then tacked down with a suture to the middle fossa floor dura. This maneuver greatly enlarges the working angle to the basilar apex. Additional details regarding aneurysm exposure and clipping will be incorporated into the specific sections on basilar apex aneurysms in Chapter 7.

■ Far Lateral Suboccipital

The far lateral suboccipital approach is a workhorse approach for exposing the inferolateral aspect of the posterior fossa. The patient can be positioned prone, three-quarter prone, or lateral. A vertical midline incision is made extending from the mid-cervical region up to the level of the inion and then curving laterally toward the mastoid process. We have generally opened the midline raphe and then cut the muscle attachments sharply from the suboccipital bone, leaving a generous cuff for reattachment. Others have preferred an incision that divides the muscles. Once the muscles have been reflected, we expose the spinous process and laminae of C2, the arch of C1, and the suboccipital bone out laterally to the mastoid tip (**Fig. 1.4**).

By working laterally along the C1 arch, the vertebral artery surrounded by its venous plexus is exposed for proximal control. The arch of C1 is removed out to the

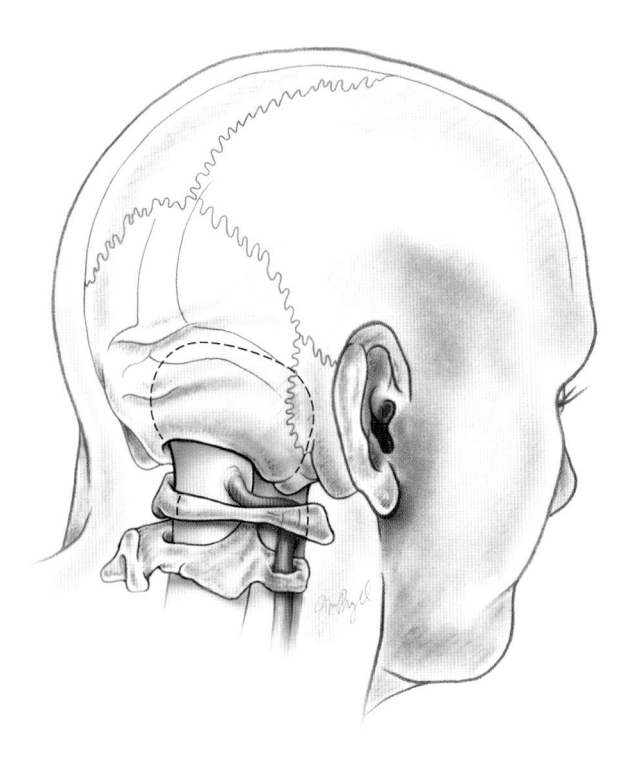

Fig. 1.4 A far lateral suboccipital approach is depicted, including the extent of bone removal (orange) of the suboccipital bone and the arch of C1. Additional bone from the condyle (green) can be removed as needed to improve visualization depending on the exact location of the lesion.

vertebral artery, and a suboccipital craniotomy is performed. In general, we bring the craniotomy just across the midline to facilitate exposure of the relevant anatomy and to offer access to the opposite posterior inferior cerebellar artery (PICA) when needed. The lateral exposure includes removal of the occipital condyle all the way out to the sigmoid region at the level of the jugular foramen. If the bone removal is done properly, the dura can be opened and reflected laterally to give a low exposure of the anterolateral brainstem, enabling visualization of the lower cranial nerves and the vertebral artery intradurally with minimal or no cerebellar retraction.

2 Aneurysms of the Anterior Cerebral Artery

■ Aneurysms of the Anterior Communicating Artery

The anterior communicating artery (ACommA) is one of the most common locations associated with intracranial aneurysm development. Although some ACommA aneurysms can be treated successfully through an endovascular approach, many are best managed with open microsurgical clipping because of a broad neck or incorporation of one of the A2 segment origins into the aneurysm base. ACommA aneurysms are generally exposed through a standard pterional approach as described in Chapter 1. We add a bit more frontal exposure for these lesions than we do for other anterior circulation aneurysms to facilitate opening of the anterior interhemispheric fissure as needed.

With the bone flap completed, the dura is elevated from the floor of the anterior cranial fossa and from the sphenoid wing. The sphenoid wing is drilled down aggressively to the region of the anterior clinoid process, and any ridges in the subfrontal bone along the superior aspect of the orbit are flattened with the drill. The periorbita is often exposed as the subfrontal bone is drilled and should be protected during this phase. By creating a low, flat plane of approach, the surgeon can limit the need for brain retraction, facilitating exposure of the aneurysm while minimizing local trauma to the brain. Once the dura has been opened, the operating microscope is introduced.

At this point, we elevate the frontal lobe gently and open the arachnoid over the optic nerve and internal carotid artery (ICA) using sharp dissection. This releases cerebrospinal fluid (CSF) and typically produces excellent brain relaxation. Traditionally, the surgeon now opens the proximal Sylvian fissure to expose the carotid bifurcation, revealing the origin of the A1 segment, which can be followed to the aneurysm. In practice, one can elevate the frontal lobe at the level of the optic nerve to identify the mid A1 segment or the aneurysm itself without first exposing the A1 origin. In our experience, when the Sylvian fissure can be opened quickly and easily, this maneuver will untether the frontal lobe and minimize the need for subfrontal retraction. When the Sylvian fissure is scarred or adherent, a very limited opening of only the most proximal aspect of the fissure will suffice in most cases.

The exact maneuvers needed to expose the aneurysm, including the degree to which the Sylvian fissure should be opened, will depend on the specific anatomical configuration of the anterior communicating complex as well as the orientation and size of the aneurysm (**Fig. 2.1**). When the aneurysm points inferiorly, one can simply elevate the frontal lobe, divide the arachnoid tethering the optic nerve to the frontal lobe, and the aneurysm will come into view (**Figs. 2.2, 2.3**) 🔄 VIDEO 1). For other configurations, it is helpful to expose and open the anterior interhemispheric fissure to visualize the A2 vessels as they exit the aneurysm 🔄 VIDEO 2). By opening the interhemispheric fissure, the surgeon can avoid gyrus rectus resection

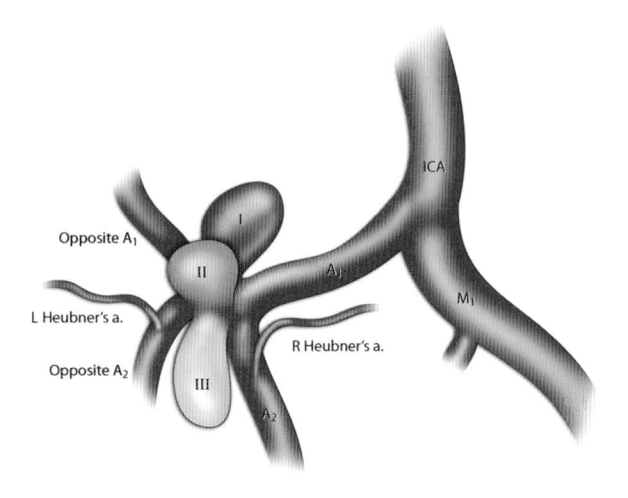

Fig. 2.1 Artist's illustration demonstrating the various typical orientations of ACommA aneurysms, which can be directed inferiorly (purple), ventrally (orange), or superiorly (yellow). A true posterior orientation is quite rare.

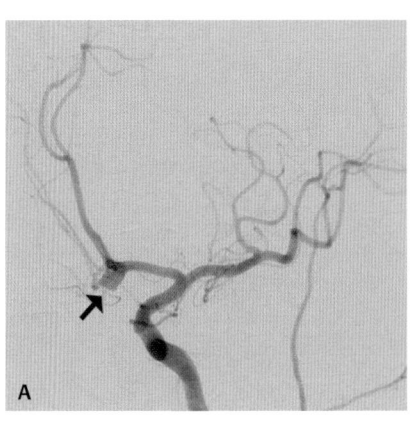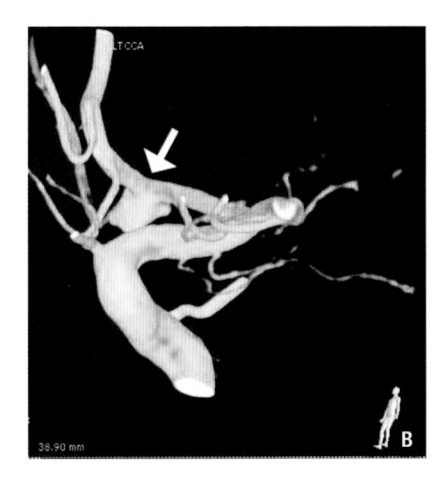

Fig. 2.2 **(A)** Oblique left internal carotid arteriogram demonstrates an inferiorly-anteriorly directed, broad-based, anterior communicating artery aneurysm (*black arrow*). **(B)** Corresponding three-dimensional rotational angiogram provides a more detailed perspective of the aneurysm arising at the junction of the left A1 and A2 segments (*white arrow*). The treatment of this lesion can be viewed in ⏵VIDEO 1.

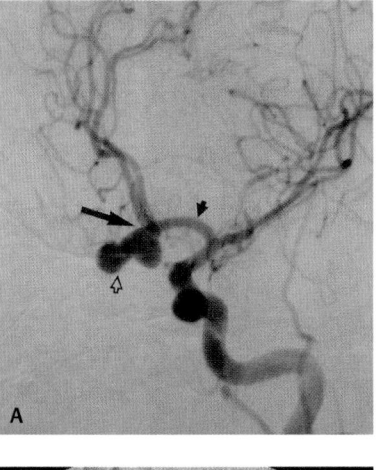

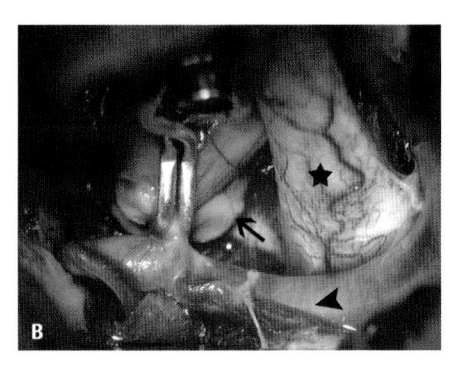

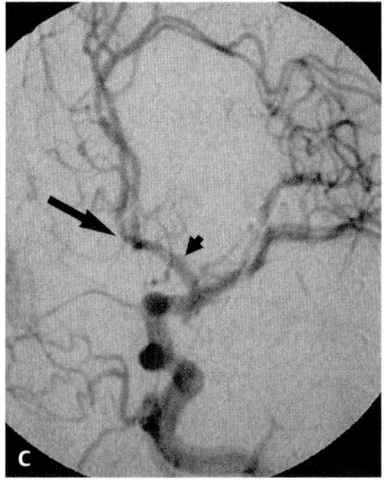

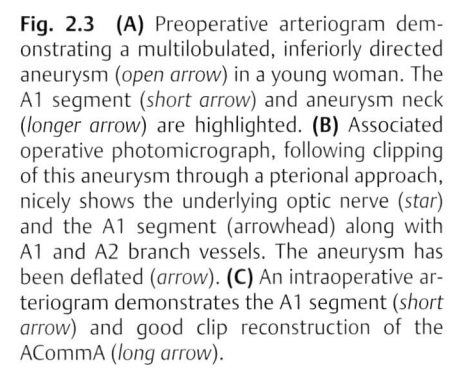

Fig. 2.3 **(A)** Preoperative arteriogram demonstrating a multilobulated, inferiorly directed aneurysm (*open arrow*) in a young woman. The A1 segment (*short arrow*) and aneurysm neck (*longer arrow*) are highlighted. **(B)** Associated operative photomicrograph, following clipping of this aneurysm through a pterional approach, nicely shows the underlying optic nerve (*star*) and the A1 segment (arrowhead) along with A1 and A2 branch vessels. The aneurysm has been deflated (*arrow*). **(C)** An intraoperative arteriogram demonstrates the A1 segment (*short arrow*) and good clip reconstruction of the ACommA (*long arrow*).

in many cases (**Fig. 2.4**). If needed, however, limited resection of the gyrus rectus can be important in exposing the key structures (**Figs. 2.5, 2.6**) VIDEO 3). In such cases, the pia is opened along an avascular area on the undersurface of the gyrus rectus, and subpial resection is then performed. Arterial branches crossing the gyrus rectus to irrigate the frontal lobe should be left intact. When the aneurysm points superiorly and posteriorly or when the ACommA rides high in the interhemispheric fissure, an orbitozygomatic (OZ) osteotomy or a more frontal exposure can be helpful.

Careful evaluation of the preoperative arteriogram should give the surgeon a good sense of the anticipated three-dimensional anatomy even before entering the

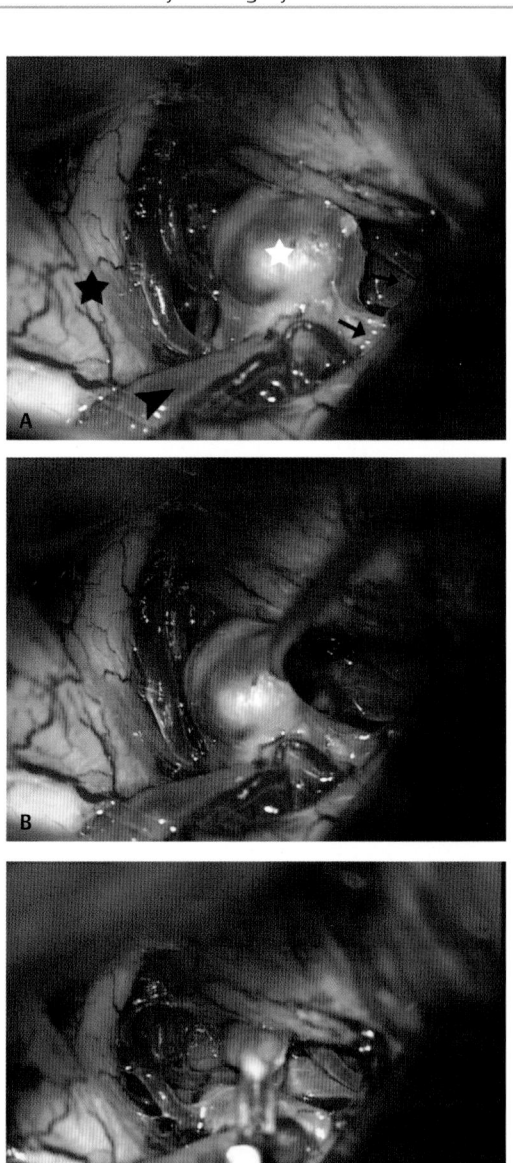

Fig. 2.4 **(A)** Operative photomicrograph reveals a broad-based, ventrally directed ACommA aneurysm (*white star*), which has been exposed by opening the anterior interhemispheric fissure to avoid resection of the gyrus rectus. Note the optic chiasm (*black star*) and nerves seen well below the aneurysm. The A1 segment (*black arrowhead*) and both A2 vessels (*small arrows*) have been exposed. **(B)** The aneurysm is then tipped forward using a dissector to expose the contralateral A2 vessel and to reveal a thin-walled component of the aneurysm directed superiorly between the A2 vessels. **(C)** The aneurysm is reconstructed with a clip, and the opposite A2 is now well visualized.

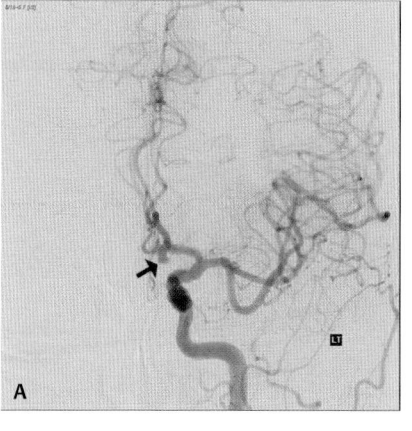

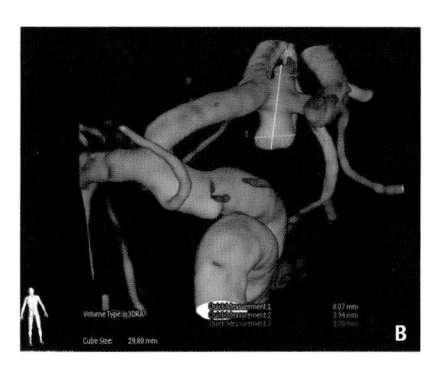

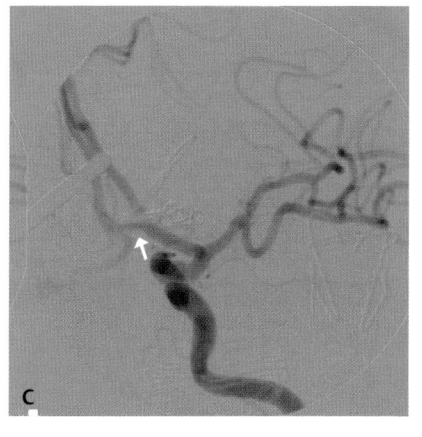

Fig. 2.5 **(A)** An anteroposterior left internal carotid arteriogram reveals a small but complex ACommA aneurysm (*black arrow*) in the setting of a recent subarachnoid hemorrhage (SAH). **(B)** A more detailed view is provided by a corresponding three-dimensional rotational angiographic study. Note the distinct inferiorly and superiorly directed components. This aneurysm is treated in 🔁 VIDEO 3 using a limited resection of the gyrus rectus. **(C)** An intraoperative angiogram demonstrates clip occlusion of the aneurysm with reconstruction of the normal ACommA (*white arrow*).

operating room (**Fig. 2.7**). It is important for the surgeon to understand the relationship of the aneurysm to the A2 vessels. As a rule, the surgeon should focus on identifying the ipsilateral and contralateral A1 vessels, the aneurysm neck, and the A2 vessels as early as possible during the surgery (**Fig. 2.8**) 🔁 VIDEO 4 🔁 VIDEO 5. Once these maneuvers are completed, proximal control can be achieved readily, and dissection of the aneurysm neck can proceed safely and with confidence. Dissection should focus on the aneurysm neck at its origin from the communicating artery, clearing a path for the tips of the clip. It is rarely necessary to dissect the entire aneurysm dome, but it may be important to free up adherent perforators to allow for proper clip placement. All perforating arteries in the region of the ACommA should be left intact. The recurrent artery of Heubner, which most commonly arises from the proximal aspect of the A2 segment and then courses back over the A1 toward the anterior perforated substance, should be identified and preserved as well.

As with all aneurysms, it is important to select a clip with properly sized blades. Overly long blades can torque the aneurysm or the normal vessels and may inadver-

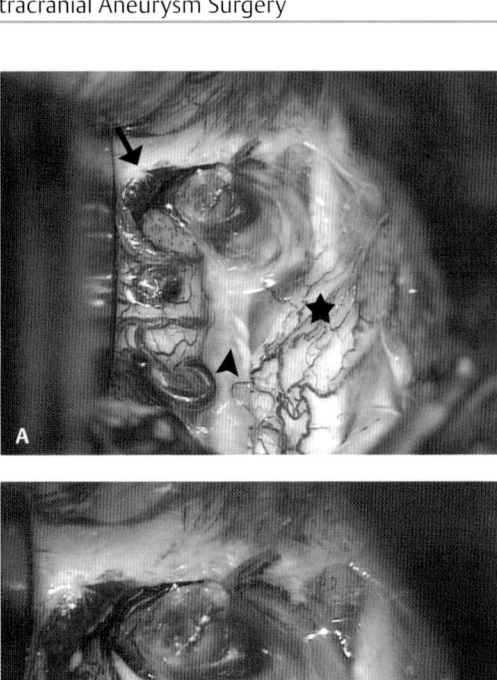

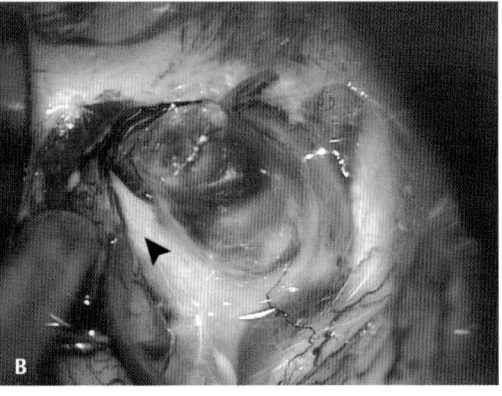

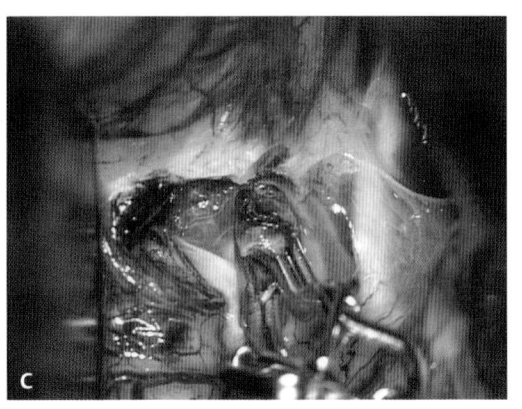

Fig. 2.6 **(A)** Operative photomicrograph demonstrating exposure of a small ruptured aneurysm of the ACommA exposed using a focal resection of the gyrus rectus (*arrow*), leaving a small amount of clot on the aneurysm dome at the site of rupture. Note the relationship of the aneurysm to the optic apparatus below (*star*). The A1 segment (*arrowhead*) has been prepared should temporary clipping be necessary. **(B)** A dissector is used to expose the aneurysm neck and its interface with the ipsilateral A2 vessel (*arrowhead*). **(C)** Two clips have been used to obliterate the aneurysm.

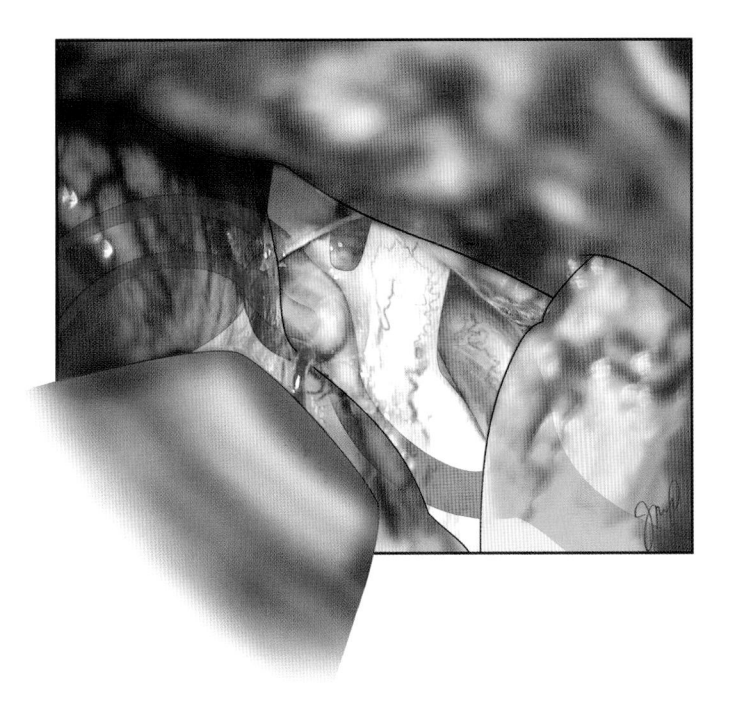

Fig. 2.7 Artist's photographic overlay illustrating an ACommA aneurysm partially hidden by the frontal lobe. Note the relationship of the A1 segment and aneurysm to the optic apparatus and overlying frontal lobe.

tently injure structures beyond the surgeon's view. Blades that are too short will fail to obliterate the aneurysm neck fully. We often find bayoneted clips to be particularly useful for ACommA aneurysms, as they allow excellent visualization of the tips of the clip as they close the aneurysm neck. When the aneurysm points superiorly and is hidden by the ipsilateral A2 vessel, a fenestrated clip can be applied with the A2 encircled in the fenestration to obliterate the aneurysm. The use of intraoperative angiography, either formal digital subtraction angiography or indocyanine green (ICG) angiography, will limit unexpected complications related to inadvertent narrowing or occlusion of a critical neurovascular structure, particularly when dealing with larger aneurysms or those with atheroma and calcification.

In the setting of a subarachnoid hemorrhage (SAH), placement of a ventriculostomy at the start of the procedure may greatly facilitate exposure of the aneurysm without undue brain retraction. We generally use a ventricular drain if there is evidence of preoperative ventriculomegaly related to a recent hemorrhage, if the brain is "full" at the start of the procedure, and in most patients who are preoperatively Hunt/Hess Grade III or higher. Although some surgeons have recommended the use of a spinal drain for unruptured lesions, we have not found this necessary, as opening of the basal CSF cisterns will generally provide excellent brain relaxation.

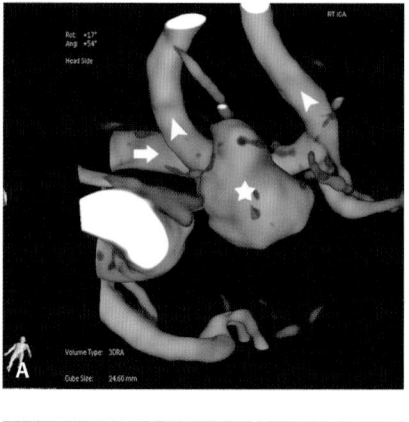

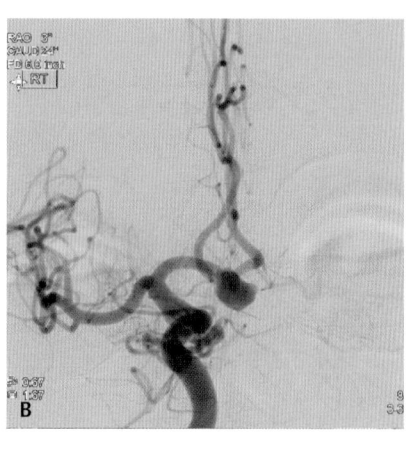

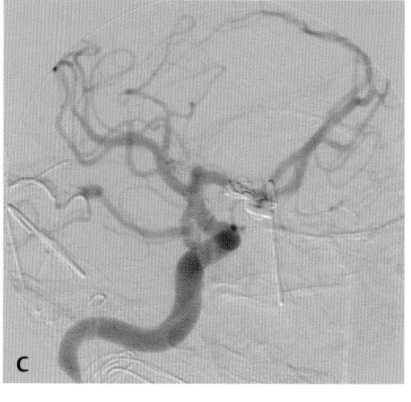

Fig. 2.8 **(A)** A three-dimensional rotational angiogram demonstrates a complex aneurysm (*star*) of the anterior communicating artery with a large, inferiorly directed lobule and a smaller ventrally directed component. The dominant A1 segment (*arrow*) and both A2 segments (*arrowheads*) are seen. **(B)** Corresponding anteroposterior right internal carotid arteriogram. This aneurysm is treated in ⏵VIDEO 4 and ⏵VIDEO 5, edited and unedited versions of the same procedure. **(C)** An intraoperative angiogram confirms obliteration of the aneurysm with preservation of the normal vasculature.

We generally approach ACommA aneurysms from the side of the dominant A1, but if the complex is rotated such that exposure of the critical anatomy would be compromised from that side, we will often use a "contralateral" approach ⏵VIDEO 6. Other mitigating factors may include the presence of additional aneurysms that can be clipped in the same setting if a particular side is chosen, a history of previous craniotomy that may make a "contralateral" approach appealing, or a large frontal hematoma from a recent hemorrhage. In this setting, it may be advisable to approach the aneurysm on the side of the hematoma to avoid injuring the preserved frontal lobe. Since the aneurysm dome will often point into the hematoma, the surgeon should always follow the basic principles already outlined, focusing attention on proximal control and working at the aneurysm neck rather than charging through the hematoma to reach the lesion. If a surgeon is working through the hematoma cavity and ruptures the aneurysm dome, it can be surprisingly disorienting and difficult to achieve proximal control without injuring critical neurovascular structures. Occasionally, a subfrontal, midline approach may be useful, although we have rarely found this necessary ⏵VIDEO 7.

Large and giant aneurysms of the ACommA are challenging because they tend to obstruct the critical vascular anatomy and can interfere with proper establishment of proximal control. In these cases, a more aggressive opening of the Sylvian and anterior interhemispheric fissures can be combined with an orbitozygomatic or orbitocranial approach and judicious resection of the gyrus rectus to expose the critical surgical anatomy properly (**Fig. 2.9**).

ACommA aneurysms are deep, midline lesions. Complications associated with their treatment generally relate to inadequate exposure of the critical anatomy,

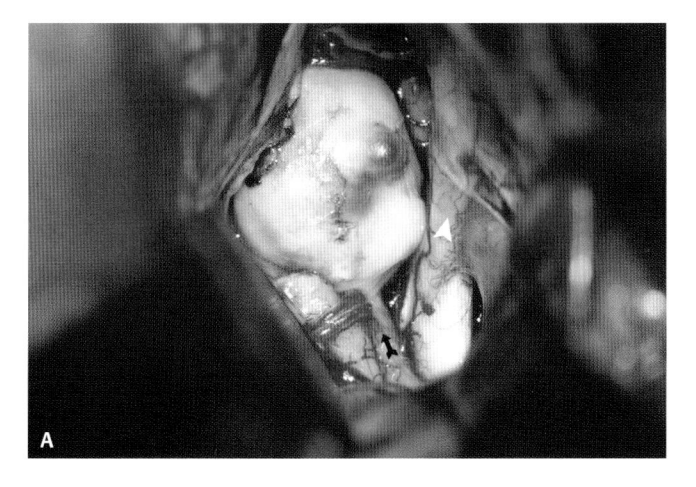

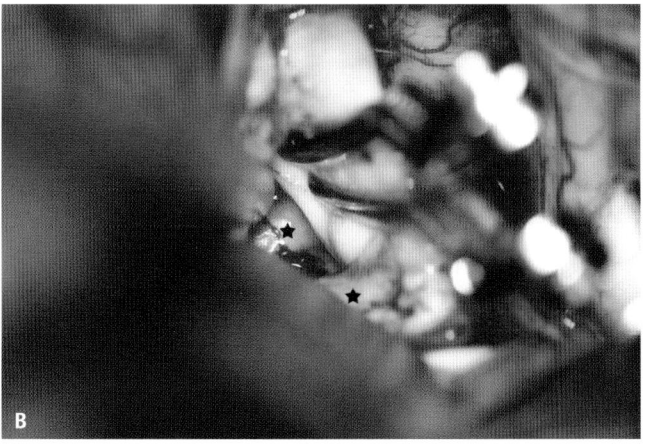

Fig. 2.9 **(A)** A large aneurysm of the ACommA has been exposed with a limited resection of the ipsilateral gyrus rectus. The A1 segment (*arrow*) and the optic nerve (*white arrowhead*) have been labeled. **(B)** The aneurysm has been tilted forward and repaired with two clips, which come just up to an atheromatous, nonfilling portion of the aneurysm along the far aneurysm neck. Excellent visualization of both A2 vessels (*stars*) is provided.

resulting in uncontrolled bleeding from a recently ruptured aneurysm or inadvertent occlusion of critical neurovascular structures. Occlusion of an anterior cerebral artery (ACA) can result in hemiparesis, particularly involving the lower extremity; temporary aphasia if the dominant supplementary motor cortex is involved; abulia and frontal lobe dysfunction; or hypothalamic/pituitary dysfunction. Severe impairment of short-term memory can be a devastating consequence of injury to the local perforating vessels and must be avoided.

The surgeon should thoroughly evaluate the preoperative imaging studies to exclude the possibility of a "third" A2 vessel, which is found in a small percentage of cases. If the surgeon is unaware of its presence preoperatively, inadvertent sacrifice of a third A2 may be missed even on intraoperative angiography as the surgeon identifies the "expected" two A2 vessels filling properly, never realizing that a third important efferent vessel has been compromised. This can result in a serious, yet completely avoidable, ischemic complication.

Because of the additional frontal exposure utilized for ACommA aneurysms, there is an increased chance of violating the frontal sinus when the bone flap is cut. In these instances, once the aneurysm has been treated, we close the dura carefully, strip the sinus mucosa, and then fill the sinus with fat harvested from the abdomen. A small amount of fat is left in the epidural space overlying the sinus opening. The patient is then maintained on an antibiotic with appropriate coverage of the sinus flora for a period of five days (**Table 2.1**).

◼ Distal ACA Aneurysms

Distal ACA aneurysms are uncommon. These lesions often present with hemorrhage. Although some are well-treated endovascularly, many have a wide neck or incorporate a major branch into the aneurysm neck, making open surgical clipping the preferred treatment. In our experience, distal ACA aneurysms have a relatively high rate of recanalization even after a successful initial coiling. As a result, despite their relative rarity, we have had the opportunity to explore and clip several previously coiled, recurrent distal ACA aneurysms.

There is great variability of the distal ACA circulation; therefore, the exact location of distal ACA aneurysms can vary considerably. Most occur at the junction between the pericallosal and callosomarginal arteries and are located near the rostrum of the corpus callosum. The exact positioning relative to the callosum can be very important in surgical decision making, as some of these aneurysms can be tucked up underneath the rostrum, making their exposure more difficult. In general, a sagittal magnetic resonance (MR) image is very helpful to assess the exact location of the aneurysm and for surgical planning. We now use frameless stereotactic guidance in these cases to help direct our approach and to limit the opening of the interhemispheric fissure and the associated dissection.

In almost all cases, distal ACA aneurysms are exposed through an interhemispheric approach via a small parasagittal craniotomy anterior to the coronal suture. The details of this approach have been outlined in Chapter 1. In general, distal ACA

Table 2.1 ■ ACommA Aneurysm Pearls and Pitfalls

Use standard pterional craniotomy with slightly more generous frontal exposure.

Use aggressive drilling of the sphenoid wing and orbital roof to create a low, flat plane of approach.

Open proximal Sylvian fissure as needed based on the local anatomy.

Open anterior interhemispheric fissure to minimize gyrus rectus trauma/removal.

OZ osteotomy may help with larger aneurysms located deep within the anterior interhemispheric fissure.

Use more aggressive opening of the fissures combined with skull base exposures for larger aneurysms.

Use a ventriculostomy in the setting of SAH when the brain is swollen to avoid injury associated with deep retraction.

Expose both A1 segments for proximal control, particularly for larger lesions.

Visualize both A2 segments for proper clip placement.

Preserve all perforating vessels.

Be sure there is not a "third" A2 vessel based on preoperative imaging.

Beware of following a hematoma cavity down to a ruptured aneurysm without first achieving proximal control and a good understanding of the critical anatomy at the neck of the aneurysm.

Superiorly/posteriorly directed lesions are the most dangerous and difficult.

Use intraoperative angiography to avoid inadvertent vascular compromise.

Evaluate A1 dominance and anatomy of the ACommA complex to choose best side for approach.

When choosing side of approach, also consider presence of additional aneurysms, history of previous craniotomy, and possible presence of frontal hematoma.

Be vigilant for inadvertent violation of the frontal sinus, which can predispose to a postoperative infection or CSF fistula.

Occlusion of an anterior cerebral artery or associated perforating vessels can result in ischemic insult with the following consequences:
• Hemiparesis (crural predominance) with possible associated aphasia
• Abulia and associated syndromes of frontal lobe dysfunction
• Hypothalamic and pituitary dysfunction (watch for diabetes insipidus)
• Severe memory impairment

aneurysms can be approached through a right-sided exposure to avoid retracting on the left hemisphere. If large draining veins are identified on the preoperative angiogram, we have used intraoperative ICG video-angiography to guide the dural opening. Interestingly, one can visualize the large veins through the intact dura, enabling precise opening of the dura without violating these venous structures. Although smaller cortical draining veins anterior to the coronal suture can usually be sacrificed without clinical consequence, we have generally avoided sacrificing any bridging veins if at all possible. This is illustrated in ⏯ VIDEO 8 . If necessary, a contralateral parasagittal bone flap can be raised in the rare event that multiple large veins hinder access to the interhemispheric fissure. It is important that the bone opening expose at least a portion of the sinus to allow for adequate access into the interhemispheric fissure. If the initial opening is found to be limiting, additional bone should be removed to expose the sinus.

Once the interhemispheric fissure has been accessed, sharp opening of the arachnoid will enable progressive deepening of the exposure. With the use of frameless stereotactic guidance, we have found that the size of our craniotomy has decreased progressively over time. It is important to remember that the surgeon will require some flexibility and working room for dissection and for clipping of the aneurysm. In fact, we have occasionally found ourselves working in a deep, narrow corridor based on a very limited opening of the interhemispheric fissure. This can limit the surgeon's ability to introduce a clip applier properly or to angle the clip blades as needed. In such circumstances, it is helpful to simply widen the opening of the interhemispheric fissure rather than trying to work in an overly confined setting.

The most critical challenge faced by the surgeon treating a distal ACA aneurysm is that of achieving proximal control. Unfortunately, the interhemispheric approach generally brings the surgeon down on the dome of the aneurysm or onto the ACAs distal to the aneurysm (**Figs. 2.10, 2.11**). Furthermore, the proximal artery feeding the aneurysm is often hidden from the surgeon's view as it curves away to run in

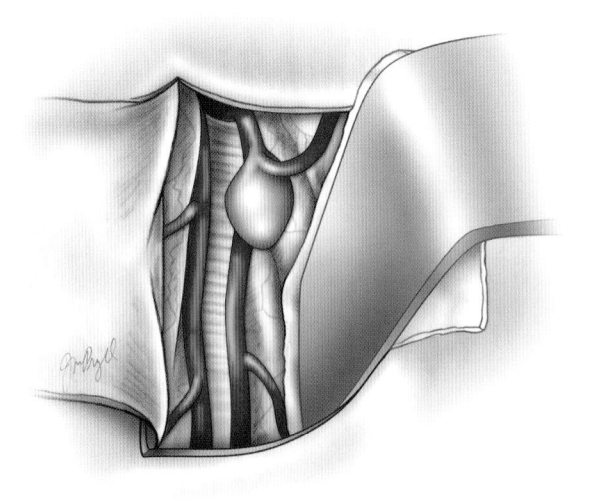

Fig. 2.10   Artist's illustration of a distal ACA aneurysm exposed through an interhemispheric approach.

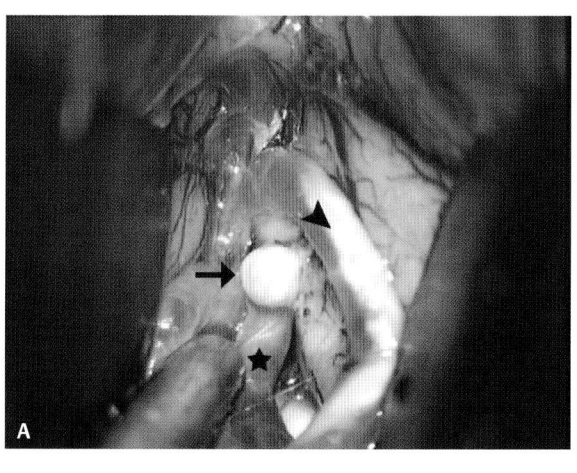

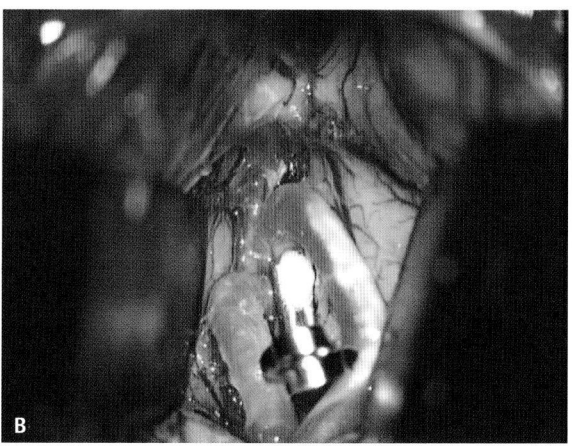

Fig. 2.11 **(A)** A distal ACA aneurysm (*arrow*) has been exposed through an interhemispheric approach. The pericallosal (*star*) and callosomarginal (*arrowhead*) arteries are seen. **(B)** The aneurysm has been repaired with a small clip.

front of the rostrum of the callosum. It is usually possible to work past the aneurysm to achieve proximal control, but in the setting of a ruptured aneurysm, the surgeon should be very careful not to overretract the hemisphere, which can put traction on the aneurysm dome and cause premature rebleeding before adequate proximal control has been achieved 🔄 VIDEO 8).

It should be noted that the dome of the aneurysm is often buried in the frontal lobe and a small amount of subpial dissection, leaving the dome attached to the pia, can be helpful to avoid premature rupture 🔄 VIDEO 9) 🔄 VIDEO 10). The surgeon must be sure to visualize all major arterial vessels prior to clip placement in this narrow working corridor. Following a severe rupture, the placement of a ventriculostomy at the start of the procedure may be helpful in obtaining brain relaxation, as the basal cisterns will not be exposed to allow for CSF drainage.

Complications associated with treating distal ACA aneurysms can result from a venous injury, arterial compromise, intraoperative aneurysm rupture, or local brain injury from excessive retraction on the medial aspect of the hemisphere. As already described, we avoid sacrificing bridging veins whenever possible to limit the risk of venous ischemia. If a vein is injured, venous hypertension can result in postoperative seizures, local brain edema, and associated subcortical hemorrhage. Distal ACA compromise can carry varying consequences depending on the degree of collateral supply. Contralateral hemiparesis, possibly associated with dysphasia, can result.

The challenge of achieving early proximal control in the setting of a distal ACA aneurysm has been described already. Severe intraoperative rupture prior to achieving proximal control can result in a significant injury; therefore, attention should be focused on achieving proximal control prior to dissection of a ruptured aneurysm. Finally, the interhemispheric approach requires retraction of the medial aspect of the hemisphere. Excessive retraction, particularly when associated with inadequate opening of the arachnoid that tethers the fissure, can result in local brain injury (**Table 2.2**).

Table 2.2　■　Distal ACA Aneurysm Pearls and Pitfalls

Frameless stereotactic guidance may be useful for approach.

Study the exact location of the aneurysm relative to the corpus callosum preoperatively.

Study preoperative arteriogram for large bridging veins when planning exposure.

Use parasagittal craniotomy, exposing at least a portion of the superior sagittal sinus.

Increase size of bone opening as needed.

Avoid sacrificing larger bridging veins—venous injury can result in venous ischemia or infarction presenting with delayed neurological deterioration, seizures, brain swelling, and hemorrhagic change.

Avoid overly narrow corridor.

Achieve proximal control as early as possible!

Avoid deep retraction prior to achieving proximal control, particularly in ruptured lesions.

If dome is adherent to frontal lobe, subpial dissection may be helpful.

Place ventriculostomy for ruptured lesions with "tight" brain.

Overly aggressive retraction on the hemisphere can lead to local injury and edema—avoid by adequately opening interhemispheric fissure.

Distal ACA occlusion can result in contralateral hemiparesis (particularly leg) or supplementary motor area syndrome.

▓ A1 Aneurysms

True aneurysms involving the A1 segment are rare. More often, aneurysms that have been described as A1 lesions are in fact ACommA aneurysms involving a fenestrated or duplicated communicating artery. Nevertheless, we have occasionally encountered aneurysms that involve the A1 segment itself. These have come in two varieties. The first group have occurred at the origin of a small perforating artery, typically arising from the medial aspect of the A1 segment. We have generally been able to clip these lesions primarily, taking care not to occlude inadvertently any perforators traversing the region toward the anterior perforated substance or optic apparatus. The second group of true A1 aneurysms have been fusiform lesions that have involved the entire circumference of the A1 artery itself. We have generally identified perforators arising directly from these lesions and have avoided primary clip reconstruction, which might sacrifice perforators in such cases. Instead, we have used proximal or distal outflow occlusion, relying on the presence of a robust contralateral A1 that fills both A2 vessels in these selected cases.

One illustrative video ⟲ VIDEO 11 ⟩ is included as a matter of interest (**Fig. 2.12**). Exposure is identical to that for anterior communicating artery aneurysms. Identification, dissection, and preservation of the recurrent artery of Heubner, as well as any A1 segment perforators adherent to the aneurysm, become critical. These aneurysms may be adherent to the optic nerve, which should be freed from the aneurysm prior to final clip placement (**Table 2.3**).

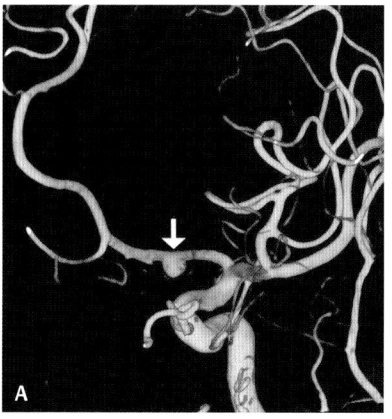
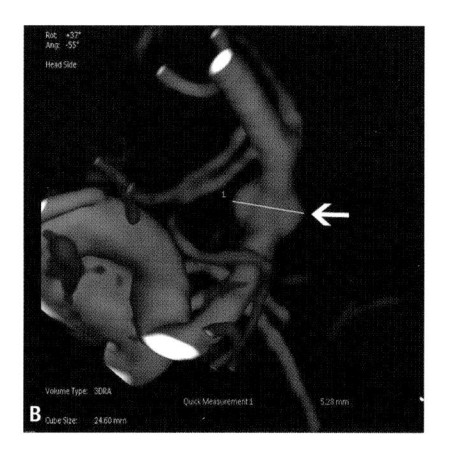

Fig. 2.12 **(A)** Three-dimensional rotational angiographic image demonstrates a rare A1 aneurysm (*white arrow*). **(B)** Magnified, rotated image demonstrates the true fusiform nature of the aneurysm (*white arrow*). This lesion is treated in ⟲ VIDEO 11 ⟩ using primary clip reconstruction.

Table 2.3 ▪ **A1 Aneurysm Pearls and Pitfalls**

These are rare lesions; treated through standard pterional craniotomy.

Expose entire A1 segment.

Identify all perforators arising from and/or traversing the A1 segment, including that of Heubner.

Separate aneurysm from optic nerve, which may be adherent to the dome.

Use primary clipping for saccular aneurysms once all perforators are identified.

Use parent artery occlusion for fusiform lesions, assuming adequate collateral from opposite A1—sacrifice of A1 should be performed only in setting of robust contra-lateral A1 with documented prompt filling of both A2's through ACommA to avoid ipsilateral A2 ischemia.

Injury to perforators may cause contralateral hemiparesis (face, arm predominance).

Perforators in region of ACommA must be preserved to avoid cognitive disturbance.

Primary or ischemic injury to optic apparatus can result in vision loss.

3 Paraclinoid Aneurysms

Paraclinoid aneurysms are common lesions. Although most are now detected at a small size, these aneurysms have a tendency to reach large and giant proportions, particularly in women. In addition, mirror image lesions are common in this location, at times complicating treatment paradigms.

From a surgical perspective, paraclinoid aneurysms can be difficult because of their intimate relationship to the anterior clinoid process, which can interfere with early establishment of proximal control (**Fig. 3.1**). These aneurysms are exposed through a standard pterional craniotomy, as described in Chapter 1, with aggressive extradural removal of the sphenoid wing. When treating a small lesion, minimal opening of the proximal Sylvian fissure, to avoid tension on the brain and bridging Sylvian veins, is usually adequate. For larger lesions, a wider opening of the fissure is helpful, and an orbitocranial (OC) approach may be useful when treating large or giant aneurysms in this location.

In our experience, in almost all cases, the anterior clinoid process must be removed at least partially and the falciform ligament opened to mobilize the optic nerve safely prior to clip placement (VIDEO 12) (VIDEO 13). The amount of clinoid removal varies depending on the local anatomy. In some cases, only a small amount of bone removal is necessary, and often the bone has been thinned already by local pressure from the aneurysm (**Figs. 3.2, 3.3**). In other instances, particularly in the setting of a short optic nerve (prefixed chiasm), we have found that a wide opening of the optic canal, at times all the way to the posterior orbit, has been necessary to allow for adequate mobilization of the optic nerve to expose the aneurysm properly without placing undue tension on the nerve itself (**Figs. 3.4, 3.5**).

As a matter of personal preference, we have favored intradural rather than extradural removal of the clinoid. In the past, we used a high-speed diamond drill for clinoidectomy. Several gently curved, fine drill bits are available that optimize the surgeon's view of the local anatomy during the drilling. For the past 5 years, we have used an ultrasonic bone-cutting device in all cases to avoid the use of a high-speed drill in close proximity to a thin-walled aneurysm. As the clinoid is removed, there is often a small amount of venous bleeding from the bone, which is readily controlled with bone wax applied using a microinstrument. Occasionally, the clinoid is highly pneumatized, and this may pose a risk for delayed cerebrospinal fluid (CSF) fistula development. In such cases, one should aggressively wax the bony opening, and we have sometimes used a small amount of muscle or fat to fill the opening at the conclusion of the procedure to avoid a delayed CSF fistula.

After removal of the clinoid, the falciform ligament is opened, and the optic nerve is freed. The aneurysm neck is then explored and the ophthalmic artery identified. On occasion, we have found the optic nerve to be densely adherent to the aneurysm dome. In such cases, the nerve can be released from under the falciform ligament and left adherent to the aneurysm dome as long as a clip can be worked

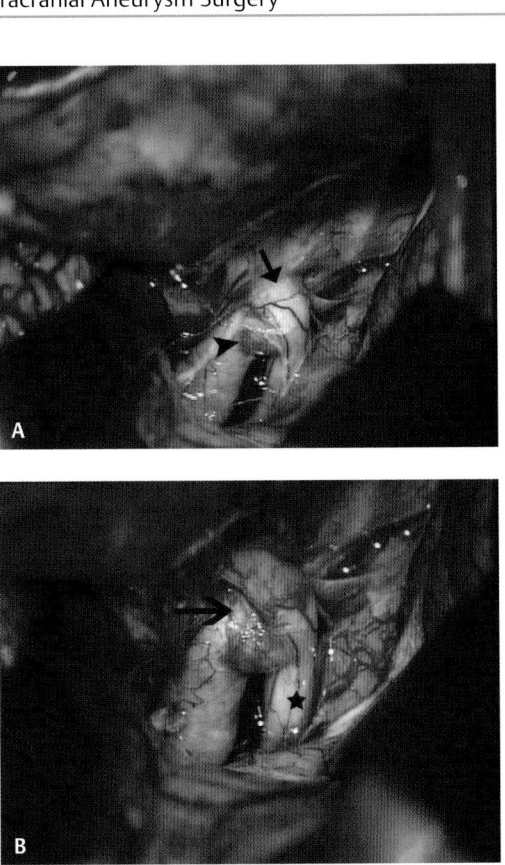

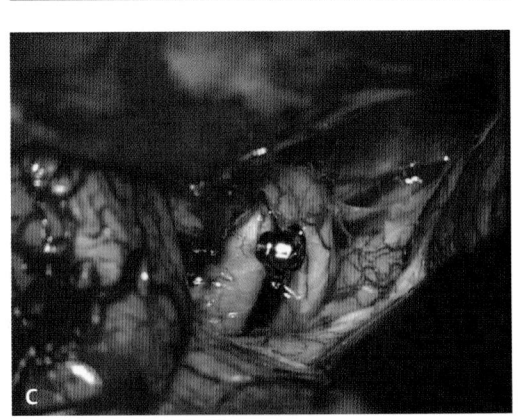

Fig. 3.1 **(A)** A left pterional craniotomy has been utilized to expose the proximal supraclinoid internal carotid artery (ICA) as well as the distal aspect of the small ophthalmic artery aneurysm (*arrowhead*), which can be seen distorting the optic nerve just proximal to the edge of the falciform ligament (*arrow*). **(B)** After a small amount of the anterior clinoid process is removed and the falciform ligament is opened, the aneurysm can be clipped without stretching the optic nerve (*star*). Note exposure of the proximal aneurysm neck and its interface with the ophthalmic artery (*arrow*). **(C)** The aneurysm has been clipped.

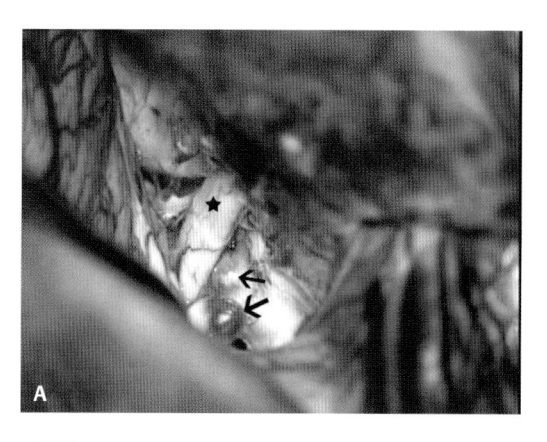

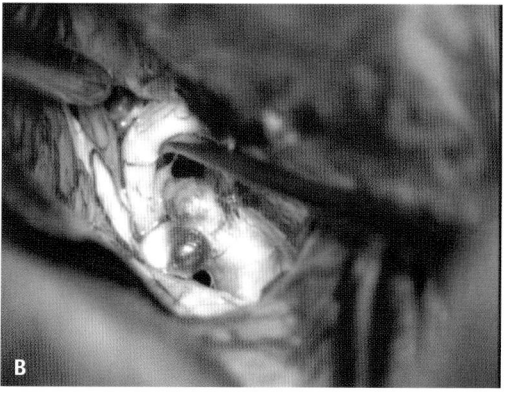

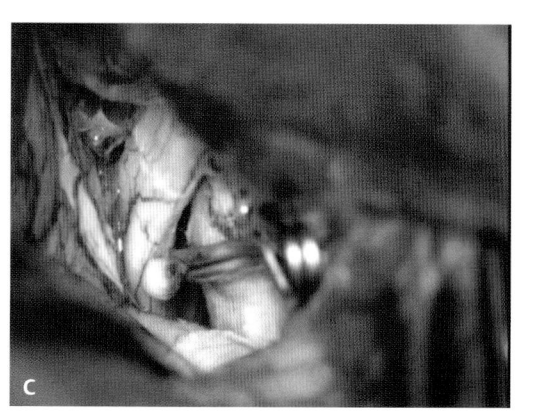

Fig. 3.2 **(A)** After removal of a small part of the anterior clinoid process and opening of the falciform ligament, this bilobed aneurysm (*arrows*) is well visualized below the optic nerve (*star*). **(B)** Gentle microdissection is used to free the aneurysms from the undersurface of the optic nerve. **(C)** A single clip is used to obliterate both lesions.

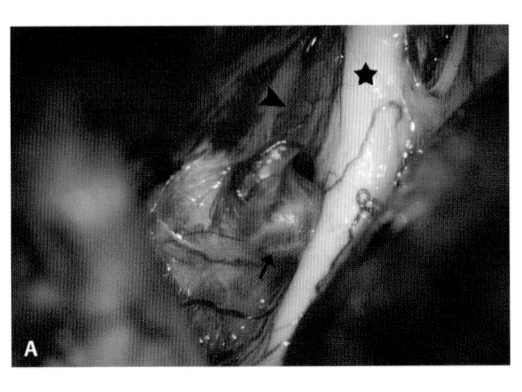

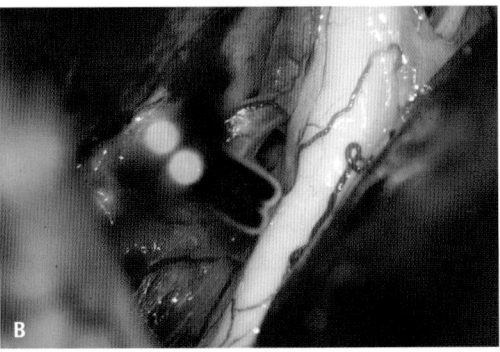

Fig. 3.3   **(A)** A tiny aneurysm (*arrow*) incorporating the origin of the ophthalmic artery (*arrowhead*) in a very young patient is exposed below the optic nerve (*star*). **(B)** The aneurysm has been repaired with a small clip, preserving the ophthalmic artery origin.

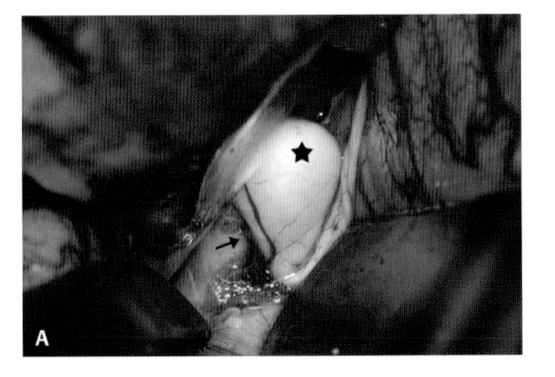

Fig. 3.4   **(A)** A pale white optic nerve (*star*) is shown stretched over the dome of a carotid ophthalmic aneurysm on initial exposure through a pterional approach. The edge of the distal aneurysm neck (*arrow*) can be seen below the nerve.

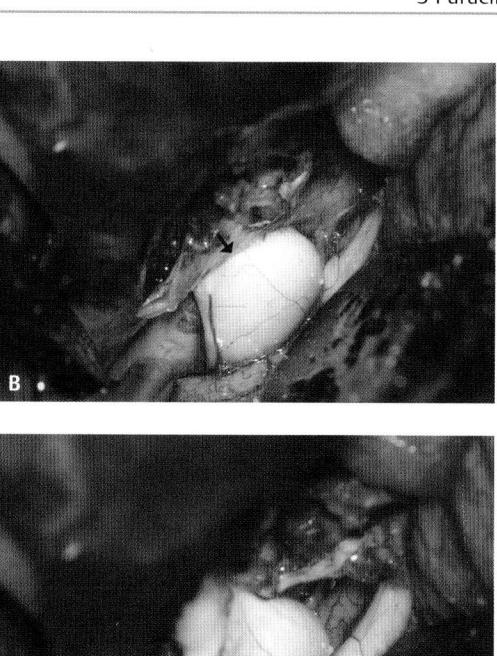

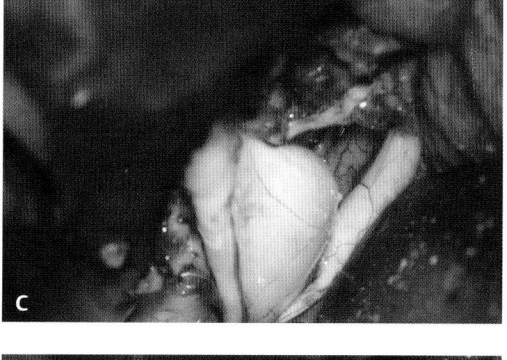

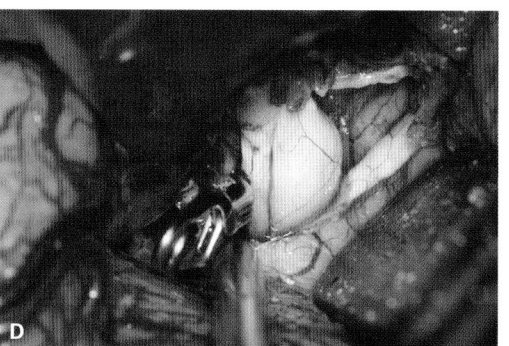

Fig. 3.4 *(Continued)*   **(B)** The dura has been opened, and the anterior clinoid process has been partially removed. The edge of the falciform ligament (*arrow*) has been left in place and still tethers the optic nerve. **(C)** The ligament has been opened and the optic nerve more fully exposed, revealing the true extent of the distortion of the nerve by the underlying aneurysm. **(D)** The aneurysm has been clipped. Note the relaxation of the nerve following repair of the underlying aneurysm.

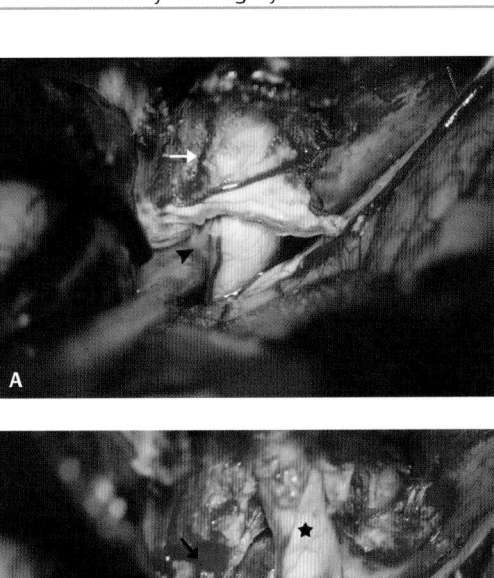

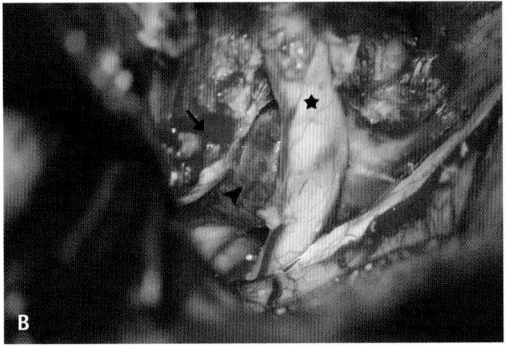

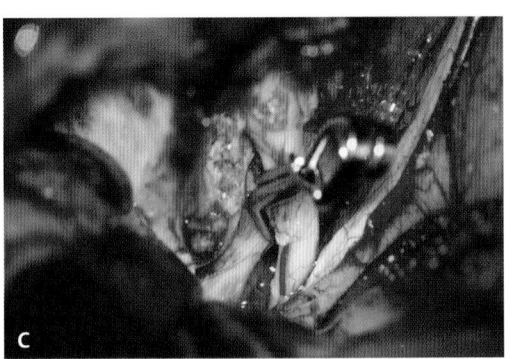

Fig. 3.5 **(A)** The dura has been opened over the anterior clinoid process, which has been partially removed (*white arrow*), leaving the falciform ligament tethering the optic nerve over the underlying aneurysm. Note how the entire aneurysm is essentially hidden from view by the stretched nerve, with only the interface between the distal neck and the ICA (*arrowhead*) visible. **(B)** Once the ligament has been opened, the optic nerve (*star*) has been freed all the way into the posterior orbit, and the broad-based underlying aneurysm (*arrowhead*) is visualized. A small amount of dural reflection (*arrow*) remains adherent to the lateral aspect of the aneurysm. **(C)** The aneurysm has been repaired with a clip, and the nerve is nicely relaxed.

across the aneurysm neck below the nerve. When treating an ophthalmic region aneurysm, visual impairment can result from overly aggressive manipulation of the optic apparatus with inadequate opening of the falciform ligament and optic canal, ischemic injury to the nerve or chiasm, occlusion of the ophthalmic artery, or thermal injury from drilling near the nerve. Following clip application, the clip itself may, on occasion, put pressure on the optic nerve or chiasm. In such cases, one can gently interpose a piece of collagen sponge material between the clip and the nerve, or a microsuture can be utilized to reposition the clip away from the optic apparatus (**Fig. 3.6**).

Paraclinoid aneurysms include a variety of anatomically distinct aneurysm subtypes. True ophthalmic aneurysms are the simplest to treat, although they require the most manipulation of the optic apparatus. Carotid cave and superior hypophyseal aneurysms require facility with skull base dissection to enable adequate exposure and clipping. It may be difficult to visualize the proximal neck of a posteriorly directed paraclinoid aneurysm, and the surgeon requires a good intuitive sense of the three-dimensional anatomy in such cases (**Fig. 3.7**) ⏺ VIDEO 14 . In all these lesions, the aneurysm dome can become intimately adherent to the basal dural reflections, which can significantly complicate the final dissection of the aneurysm. In addition, it may be difficult to predict which aneurysms are partially extradural, and complete clipping may require opening of the proximal and distal dural rings of the cavernous sinus. Bleeding from the cavernous sinus can be bothersome, and surgeons treating these lesions should be comfortable with this possibility.

Large and giant aneurysms in this location are more difficult because of their distortion and compression of the optic apparatus ⏺ VIDEO 15 (**Fig. 3.8**). Options for proximal control include exposure of the cervical internal carotid artery (ICA) through a neck incision, the use of a balloon microcatheter positioned endovascu-

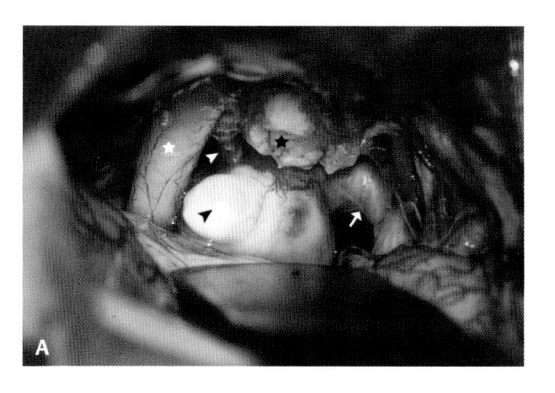

Fig. 3.6 **(A)** A large ophthalmic-region aneurysm has been exposed by opening the falciform ligament after partial removal of the anterior clinoid process (*black star*). The optic nerve (*white star*) is displaced medially by a heavily atheromatous, nonfilling portion of the aneurysm (black arrowhead). The ICA (*white arrow*) and the ophthalmic artery (*white arrowhead*) are seen. (*Continued on page 32*)

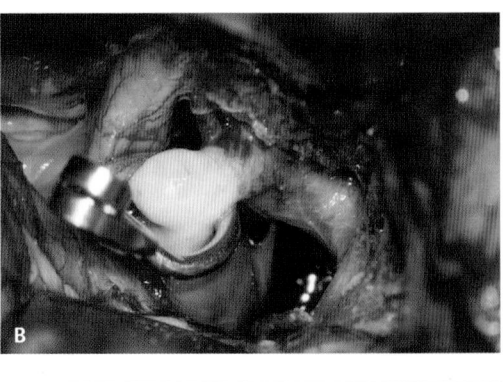

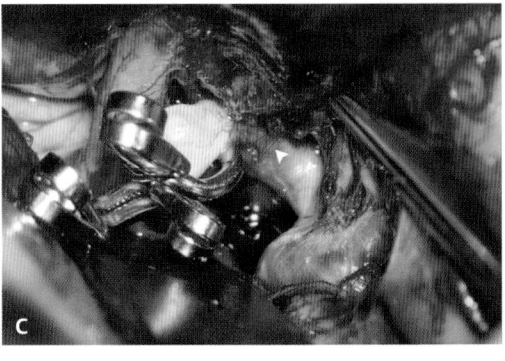

Fig. 3.6 *(Continued)*   **(B)** A fenestrated clip has been used to repair the aneurysm, leaving the atheromatous, nonfilling potion of the aneurysm open in the fenestration, as a simple clip would not close because of the calcification in the wall. Note how the medial aspect of the fenestration indents the optic nerve. **(C)** A 10-0 microsuture (*white arrow*) has been used to pull the clip away from the optic apparatus by suturing the clip down to the basal dura.

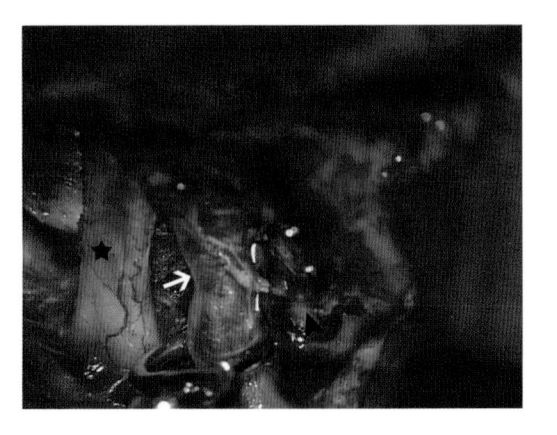

Fig. 3.7   A proximal paraclinoid aneurysm (*black arrowhead*) has been clipped using an an-gled fenestrated clip around the ICA (*white arrow*). The optic nerve is seen as well (*black star*).

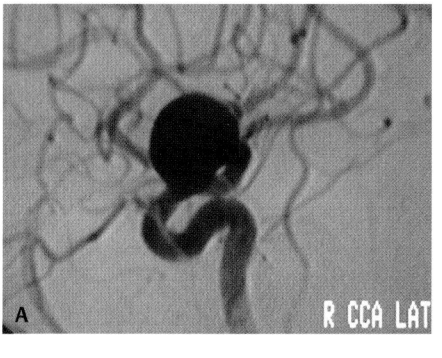
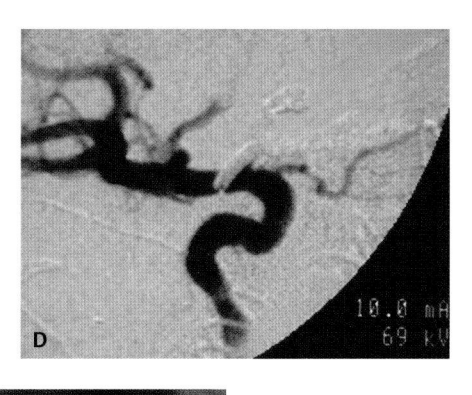
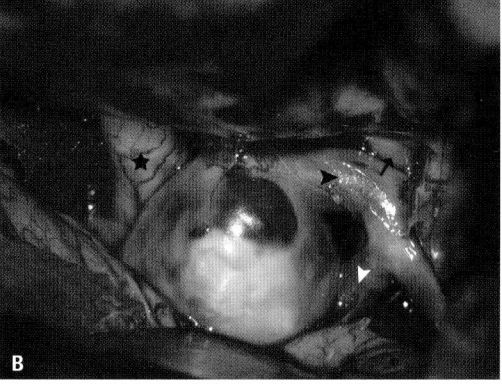
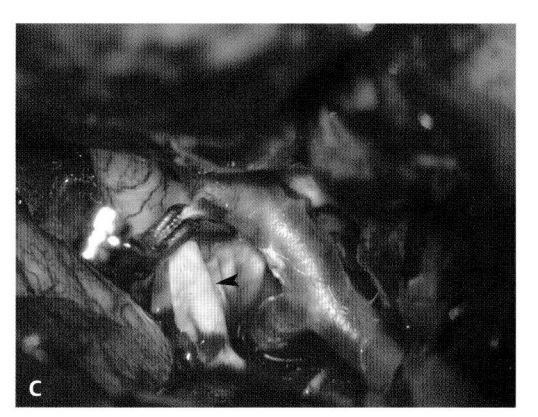

Fig. 3.8 **(A)** A lateral internal carotid arteriogram reveals a large paraclinoid aneurysm in a young woman with visual disturbance. **(B)** The aneurysm has been exposed through a pterional approach, revealing the optic nerve (*star*), supraclinoid ICA (*arrowhead*), and third cranial nerve (*arrow*). **(C)** The aneurysm has been clipped and deflated (*arrowhead*) to decompress the optic nerve. **(D)** Postoperative angiography reveals occlusion of the aneurysm. This lesion is treated in ⏵ VIDEO 15 .

larly in the cervical ICA, or exposure of the petrocavernous carotid through a complex skull base dissection. When treating giant paraclinoid aneurysms, we generally expose the cervical ICA for possible suction decompression of the aneurysm. The endovascular placement of a balloon in the cervical internal carotid artery represents a reasonable alternative, although we have found it faster and more reliable to primarily expose the cervical carotid artery. The use of an endovascular balloon for any period of time carries a thromboembolic risk, and repeated inflation and deflation of the balloon can result in a carotid dissection. In addition, we have occasionally had trouble achieving adequate decompression with a balloon. When using suction decompression, it is important to apply a clip distal to the aneurysm across the supraclinoid internal carotid artery prior to beginning the suction to avoid stealing important collateral flow from the ipsilateral hemisphere. Despite temporary occlusion and suction decompression, giant paraclinoid lesions can be very challenging to clip when densely adherent to the basal dura or the optic apparatus. Examples of giant paraclinoid aneurysms treated with direct clip reconstruction and with bypass and occlusion are included in Chapter 9.

When treating a ruptured paraclinoid aneurysm, the issue of proximal control becomes even more critical. In the setting of a severe, unexpected intraoperative rupture of a carotid ophthalmic aneurysm, we have used an intravenous infusion of adenosine to induce transient cardiac standstill, providing temporary flow arrest when proximal control could not be achieved easily. Note that bilateral ophthalmic aneurysms, when small, can often be clipped via a unilateral approach, dissecting and clipping the contralateral aneurysm by working underneath the opposite optic nerve (**Fig. 3.9**) (**Table 3.1**).

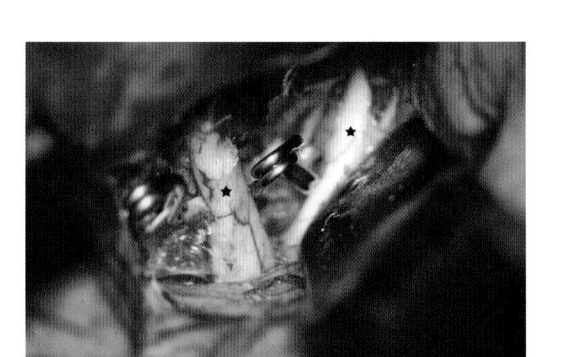

Fig. 3.9 A left pterional craniotomy has been performed, and bilateral small ophthalmic region aneurysms have been exposed and clipped by opening the falciform ligaments to mobilize the optic nerves (*stars*) bilaterally.

Table 3.1 ▪ **Paraclinoid Aneurysm Pearls and Pitfalls**

Use standard pterional craniotomy with limited opening of proximal Sylvian fissure.

Use aggressive drilling of the sphenoid wing and orbital roof to create a low, flat plane of approach.

Use a wider Sylvian opening and possible orbitocranial approach for larger and giant aneurysms.

Proximal control may be hindered by the anterior clinoid process hiding the proximal aneurysm neck and proximal ICA.

Remove the clinoid and open the falciform ligament to enable optic nerve mobilization.

Consider cervical ICA exposure or endovascular balloon placement in cervical ICA for large or giant aneurysms.

Identify and protect the ophthalmic artery itself.

The aneurysm neck must be fully exposed and freed prior to clip placement.

When using suction decompression, be sure to apply distal clip to supraclinoid ICA prior to suction.

Remember that the external carotid artery (ECA) may supply collaterals via the ophthalmic artery, preventing adequate decompression or resulting in ongoing bleeding if aneurysm ruptures intraoperatively.

Contralateral paraclinoid aneurysms can usually be treated at the same setting, particularly when small.

Large and giant aneurysms may be adherent to the optic apparatus and basal dura and may defy primary clipping attempts.

Visual impairment can result from:
• Overly aggressive manipulation of optic apparatus without adequate opening of falciform ligament and optic canal
• Ischemic injury to nerve or chiasm or occlusion of ophthalmic artery itself
• Thermal injury from drilling near nerve

Carotid occlusion or stenosis may result in hemispheric ischemic insult, depending on adequacy of collateral circulation.

Unrecognized opening of pneumatized anterior clinoid process can predispose to delayed CSF fistula and/or infection.

4 Supraclinoid Internal Carotid Artery Aneurysms

The majority of aneurysms involving the supraclinoid internal carotid artery (ICA) arise at the origins of the posterior communicating or anterior choroidal arteries. We will address aneurysms arising at these locations individually. In addition, over the past decade, increasing recognition has been given to a unique subset of aneurysms involving the ventral supraclinoid ICA not associated with a clear branch point or perforating vessel. These lesions are often dissecting aneurysms. They tend to have a highly malignant natural history and can be extremely unstable.

A pterional craniotomy is utilized for the treatment of aneurysms involving the supraclinoid portion of the ICA. For lesions arising at the origins of the posterior communicating or anterior choroidal arteries, the Sylvian fissure need be opened only to the level of the carotid bifurcation. In most cases, proximal control is readily achieved. We will discuss the management of ventral supraclinoid aneurysms as a separate entity.

■ Posterior Communicating Artery Aneurysms

Posterior communicating artery (PCommA) aneurysms have traditionally been thought of as "easy" aneurysms from a surgical perspective. In academic training programs, these lesions have often been considered reasonable fodder for mid-level residents yearning to clip their first aneurysms. In our experience, there is great variability in the difficulty associated with these lesions. Although most will be visible immediately upon opening the arachnoid lateral to the ICA just above the level of the optic nerve, these aneurysms can sometimes be obscured from view by a large anterior clinoid process, which can also compromise early establishment of proximal control (**Figs. 4.1, 4.2**). In addition, when the supraclinoid ICA itself is short or lies in a very horizontal orientation, the aneurysm may point deeply away from the surgeon during a routine pterional exposure. Most often, however, these lesions are well exposed through a standard pterional approach.

Much has been written about proper patient positioning when treating a ruptured PCommA aneurysm based on whether or not the patient presents with a third-nerve palsy. In general, if the patient does not have a third-nerve palsy, then the aneurysm is suspected to be directed laterally, where its dome can adhere to the temporal lobe. In such cases, too much rotation of the head can encourage the surgeon to utilize aggressive temporal lobe retraction, which can cause the aneurysm to rebleed. In our experience, it is best to avoid deep temporal retraction in all PCommA aneurysms, and a standard pterional approach with the head turned no more than 45 degrees works best in such cases. By opening the proximal Sylvian fissure, the surgeon can identify the neck of the aneurysm first, and a small bit of

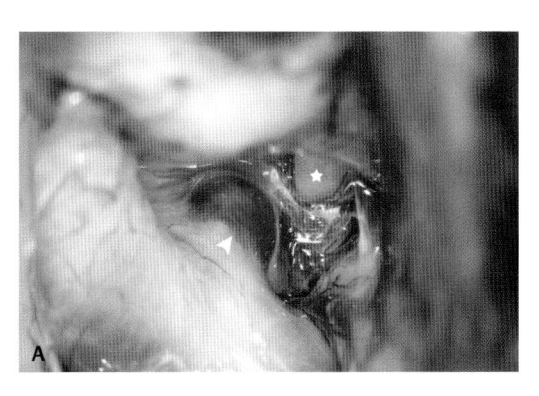

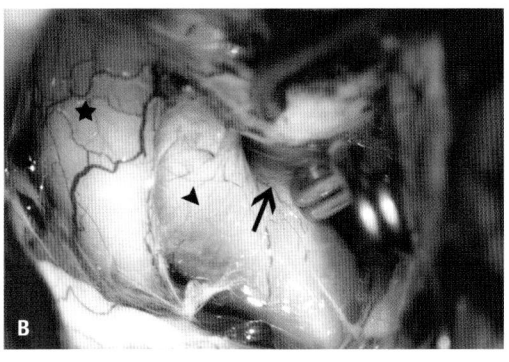

Fig. 4.1 **(A)** A small, very thin-walled PCommA aneurysm (*arrowhead*) on the right side is visualized through a pterional approach. Note the proximity to the third cranial nerve (*star*). **(B)** The aneurysm has been repaired with a clip. The optic nerve (*star*) and the proximal ICA (*arrowhead*) are seen. Note the normal PCommA origin (*arrow*), which is visible between the clip and the parent ICA.

subpial resection can be used to free the aneurysm dome if necessary prior to clip placement. This maneuver avoids any traction being placed on the deep temporal lobe, which can, in theory, result in tearing of the aneurysm.

For all PCommA aneurysms, the proximal Sylvian fissure should be opened sharply, exposing the supraclinoid ICA at the level of the optic nerve ⏩ VIDEO 16 ⏩ VIDEO 17). This maneuver will establish proximal control in most cases. Depending on the size of the aneurysm, the surgeon will have to address both the PCommA itself as well as the neighboring anterior choroidal artery (AChA). The PCommA should be identified and its origin preserved (**Fig. 4.3**). In some cases, the neck of the aneurysm may incorporate the origin of the artery, and a carefully placed clip will enable the reconstruction of the origin of the PCommA. In rare cases, when the PCommA origin is incorporated into the aneurysm neck and there is clear filling of the posterior cerebral artery (PCA) and the PCommA itself in retrograde fashion from the basilar artery, the PCommA origin can be occluded along with the

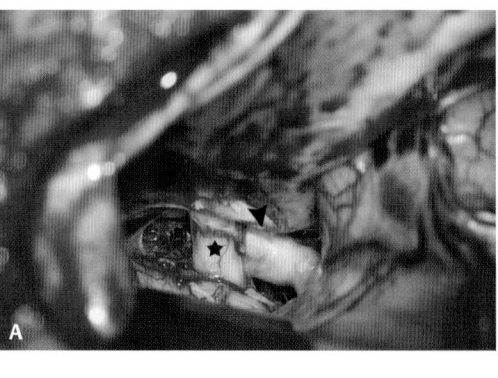

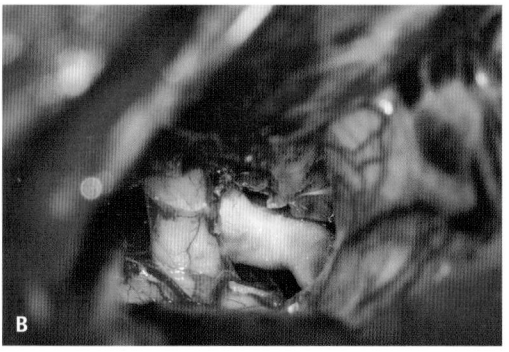

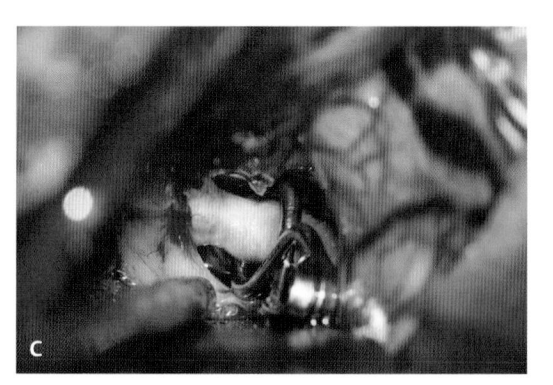

Fig. 4.2 **(A)** A right pterional craniotomy has been performed and the proximal supraclinoid ICA and the optic nerve (*star*) have been exposed. The PCommA aneurysm is not visible because of the large anterior clinoid process (*arrowhead*) and the horizontal orientation of the internal carotid artery. **(B)** A portion of the clinoid has been removed to allow for exposure of the aneurysm. **(C)** The aneurysm has been repaired with a fenestrated clip encircling the ICA.

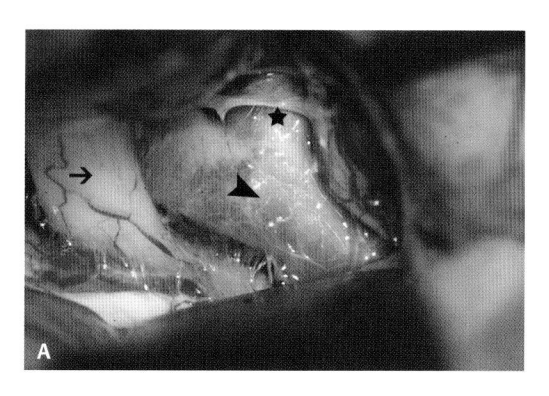

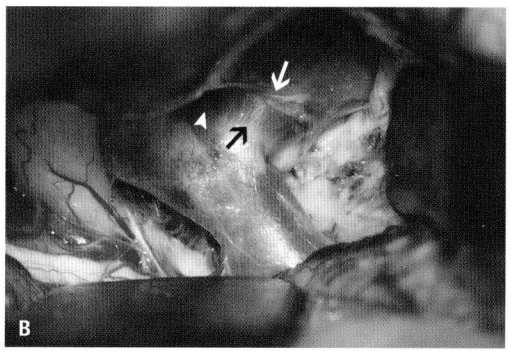

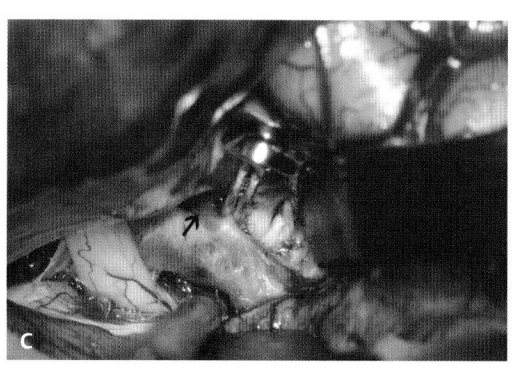

Fig. 4.3 **(A)** A pterional craniotomy has been performed to expose the neck (*star*) of a large PCommA aneurysm. The optic nerve (*arrow*) and supraclinoid ICA (*arrowhead*) are seen. **(B)** The true neck of the aneurysm (*arrow*) and the origin of the PCommA (*white arrowhead*) are now visible. Note how most of the aneurysm is hidden below the edge of the tentorium (*white arrow*). **(C)** The aneurysm has been clipped, and the large PCommA origin is visible (*arrow*) proximal to the clip.

aneurysm neck. In these very rare cases, we always check an intraoperative vertebral arteriogram to be sure the PCA as well as the PCommA both fill promptly. The PCommA typically gives rise to critical anterior thalamoperforating vessels, and these can be injured by overly long clip blades reaching past the aneurysm neck toward the perimesencephalic cistern.

Before operating on a PCommA aneurysm, it is important to understand the anatomy of the ipsilateral PCA based on preoperative angiography (**Fig. 4.4**). If the PCommA represents a fetal PCA (i.e., the ipsilateral P1 is atretic), then occlusion or stenosis of the PCommA can result in a serious PCA infarction with complete hemianopsia. Ischemic injury due to loss of the anterior thalamoperforators can further complicate the situation. As a result, one should not sacrifice a fetal PCommA.

If the AChA is adherent to or running along the aneurysm dome, it must be thoroughly dissected away, at least from the aneurysm neck, prior to clip placement. AChA occlusion can result in contralateral hemiparesis, hemisensory loss, and hemianopsia, and such occlusion should be avoided in all situations (**Fig. 4.5**) ⏯ VIDEO 18).

PCommA aneurysms are situated close to the third cranial nerve. An expanding PCommA aneurysm can result in partial or complete third-nerve palsy, a situation

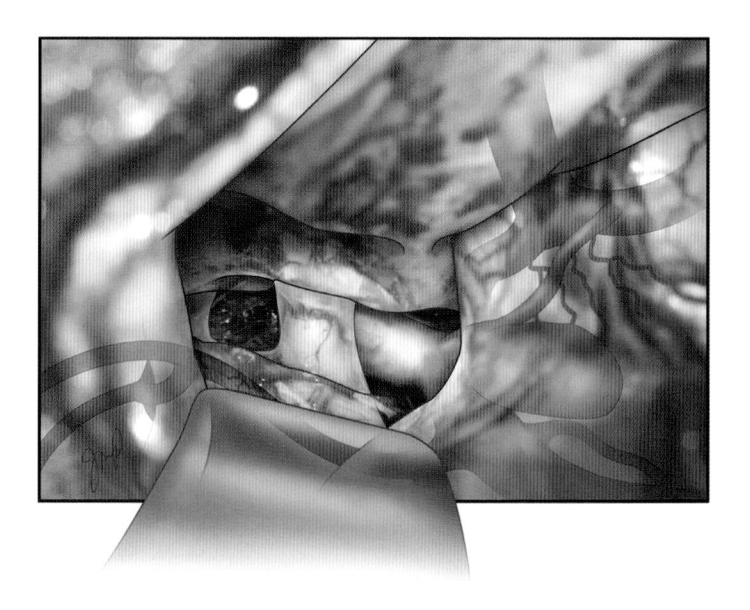

Fig. 4.4 Artist's overlay rendering illustrates the positioning of a PCommA aneurysm prior to opening of the proximal Sylvian fissure. Note the extent to which the fissure must be opened to expose the proximal and distal neck of the aneurysm.

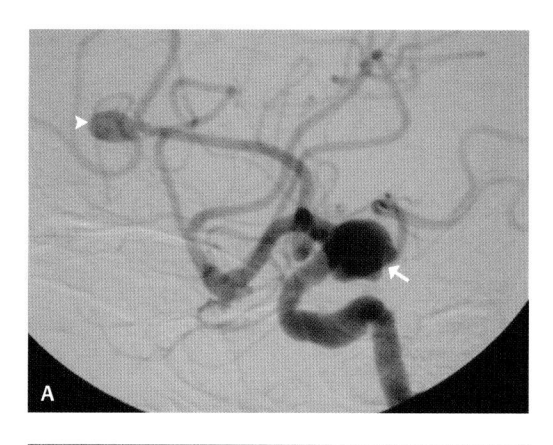

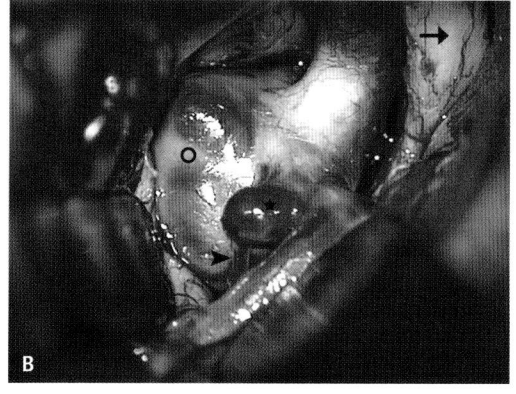

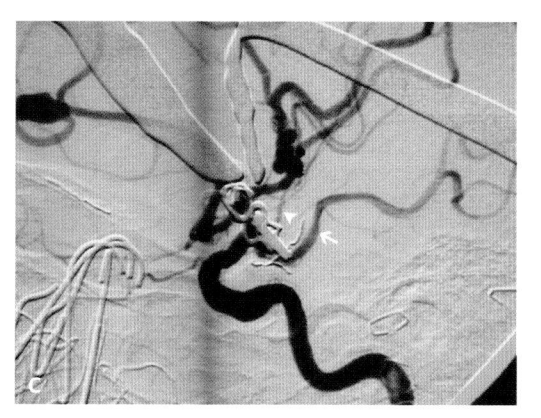

Fig. 4.5 **(A)** A lateral preoperative internal carotid arteriogram demonstrates a large aneurysm (*arrow*) of the PCommA as well as a distal ACA aneurysm (*arrowhead*). **(B)** Operative photomicrograph reveals the large posterior communicating region aneurysm (*circle*) as well as a smaller anterior choroidal aneurysm (*star*) with the AChA (*arrowhead*) sandwiched between the two aneurysms. The optic nerve is identified as well (*arrow*). **(C)** An intraoperative angiogram demonstrates good clip reconstruction of the aneurysms with preservation of the PCommA (*arrow*) and AChA (*arrowhead*). This surgical procedure is shown in 🔁 VIDEO 17). The incidentally noted distal ACA aneurysm was clipped in a subsequent surgery.

that should generally be treated with urgent repair of the aneurysm before a life-threatening subarachnoid hemorrhage (SAH) occurs (**Fig. 4.6**). There is some controversy as to whether open surgery or endovascular coiling should be performed in this setting. In our experience, the third-nerve palsy tends to improve in the majority of cases treated in either fashion, although there may be a slight advantage to open surgery, which enables immediate deflation of the aneurysm and decompression of the nerve.

When PCommA aneurysms become large, they can become more difficult to treat using simple neck clipping. One important surgical strategy involves the use of fenestrated clips, often with right-angle blades, placed around the ICA to occlude the aneurysm neck (**Fig. 4.7**). In these cases, one must be particularly careful to avoid compromising the origin of the AChA.

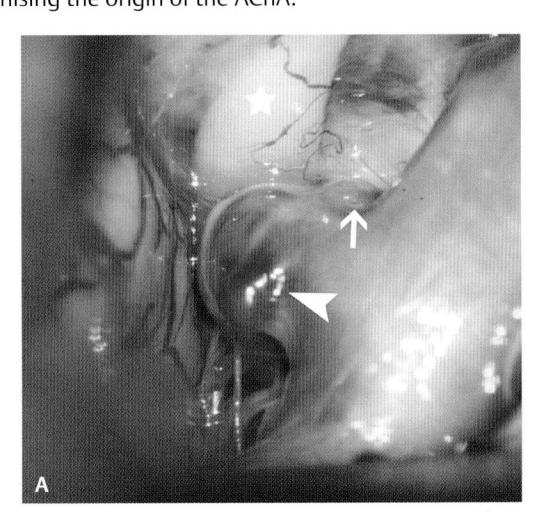

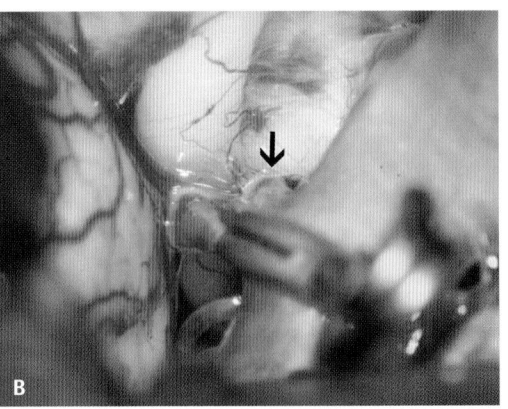

Fig. 4.6 **(A)** A small posterior communicating artery aneurysm presenting with a partial third-nerve palsy is exposed. Note the thin blister-like area (*arrowhead*) at the aneurysm base, the origin of the PCommA (*arrow*), and the proximity to the third cranial nerve (*star*). **(B)** The aneurysm has been clipped, preserving the PCommA origin (*arrow*).

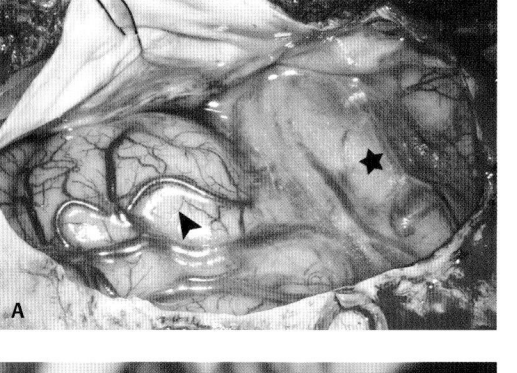

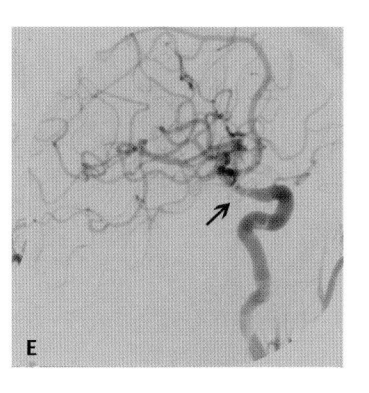

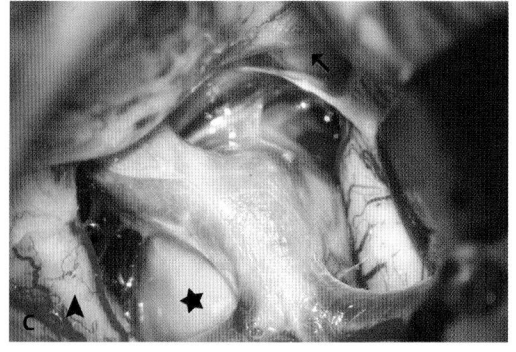

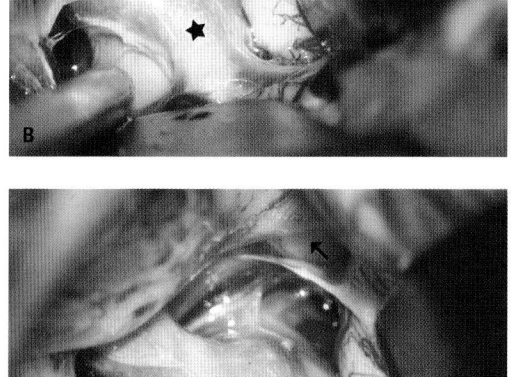

Fig. 4.7 **(A)** A pterional craniotomy has been performed, revealing the frontal (*arrowhead*) and temporal (*star*) lobes. **(B)** The proximal Sylvian fissure has been opened to expose a giant, partially thrombosed aneurysm of the PCommA. A portion of the aneurysm is seen as a whitish gray structure underneath the suction tip and behind the supraclinoid ICA (*star*). **(C)** A more magnified view reveals the aneurysm (*star*), the optic nerve (*arrowhead*), and the third nerve (*arrow*). **(D)** The aneurysm has been reconstructed using a right-angled fenestrated clip applied around the internal carotid artery. Note how the aneurysm dome is beginning to turn blue. **(E)** An intraoperative angiogram demonstrates reconstruction of the supraclinoid ICA (*arrow*) without residual filling of the aneurysm.

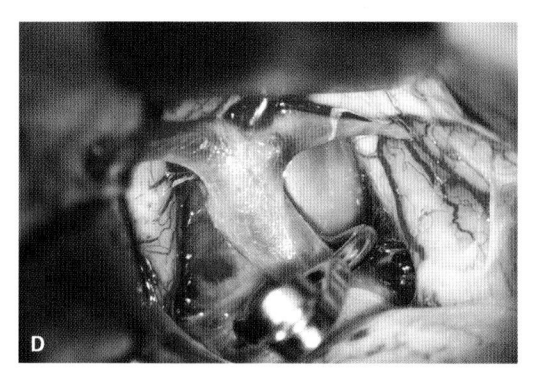

Finally, PCommA aneurysms will occasionally present with a large temporal lobe hematoma or a subdural hematoma, resulting in a life-threatening herniation syndrome. A preoperative CT scan with contrast will often show the underlying aneurysm in such cases, and the patient is brought to the operating room on an emergency basis without a formal preoperative arteriogram. A generous craniotomy is performed to enable decompression, and then an intraoperative angiogram is performed to assess the neurovascular anatomy. In general, one can evacuate some of the hematoma to decompress the brain without rupturing the aneurysm. In these cases, we prefer to open the proximal Sylvian fissure, expose the aneurysm neck, and clip the aneurysm in standard fashion, rather than working through the hematoma cavity to reach the aneurysm. Once the aneurysm has been clipped, remaining hematoma is removed, and a decision can be made whether the bone flap can be replaced safely or whether the degree of brain swelling mandates that the flap be temporarily stored for later re-implantation (**Table 4.1**).

Table 4.1   ■   Posterior Communicating Artery Aneurysm Pearls and Pitfalls

Use standard pterional craniotomy; avoid turning the head more than 45 degrees.

Use aggressive drilling of the sphenoid wing and orbital roof to create a low, flat plane of approach.

Open proximal Sylvian fissure sharply to expose the supraclinoid ICA at the level of the optic nerve for proximal control.

Not all PCommA aneurysms are simple; proximal control can be an issue in patients with very short and horizontal supraclinoid ICA segments.

The AChA and PCommA should be identified and preserved.

The PCommA gives rise to critical thalamoperforating arteries.

The PCommA should never be sacrificed unless one is absolutely sure there is a healthy P1 segment that fills the distal PCA and PCommA.

A fenestrated clip can be used to reconstruct the ICA in larger lesions, but watch the AChA origin.

Identify the origin of the AChA and free the AChA from the aneurysm neck as needed.

Subpial resection along aneurysm dome may be preferable to deep temporal lobe retraction if dome must be freed for proper clip placement.

Beware of following a hematoma cavity down to a ruptured aneurysm without first achieving proximal control and a good understanding of the critical anatomy at the neck of the aneurysm.

Occlusion of the PCommA can result in a PCA infarct with anterior thalmoperforating injury as well.

Occlusion of the AChA can result in contralateral hemiparesis, hemisensory loss, and hemianopsia.

■ Anterior Choroidal Artery Aneurysms

Aneurysms arising at the origin of the AChA are typically small and often confused with PCommA aneurysms on initial angiographic review. In fact, the complication rates associated with AChA aneurysms are high, probably because of frequent injury to the AChA itself or to one of its fine branches during surgery. In our experience, the AChA is often duplicated or gives rise to multiple branches, which may run along the aneurysm dome and are prone to injury during clipping (**Fig. 4.8**). We have included video of a case that illustrates the duplication of the AChA in association with an aneurysm VIDEO 19 .

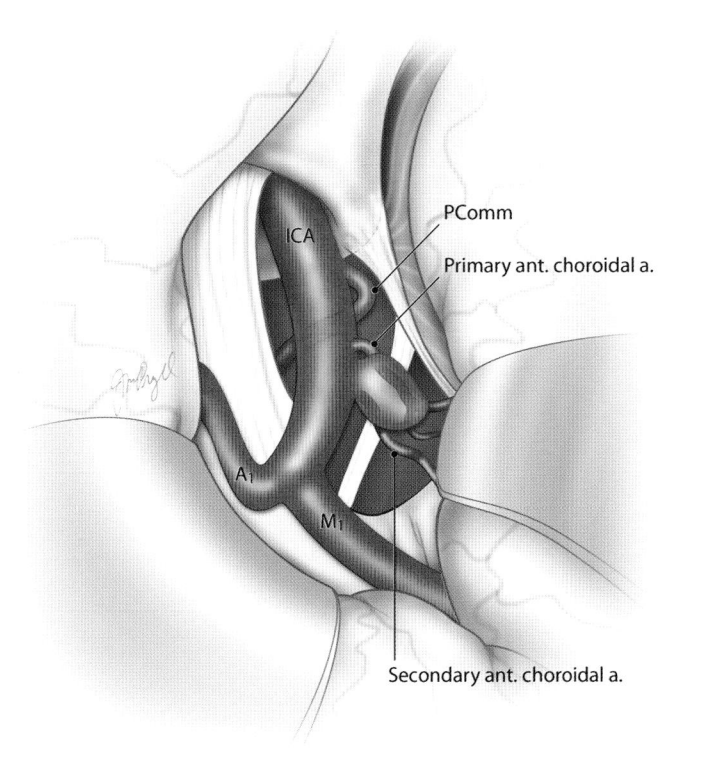

Fig. 4.8   Artist's illustration demonstrating the duplicated and branching nature of the anterior choroidal vasculature, which is often hidden from the surgeon's view behind the aneurysm itself and is therefore prone to inadvertent injury during clipping.

These aneurysms are exposed and treated via a pterional craniotomy following the protocol outlined above for posterior communicating aneurysms (VIDEO 20) (**Fig. 4.9**). The surgeon must meticulously dissect the AChA, any accessory choroidal artery, and all branches from the aneurysm neck to apply a clip safely (**Figs. 4.10, 4.11**). Intraoperative angiography is critical in these cases to ensure that the AChA is filling properly after clip placement. Although neurosurgeons are quick to point out that surgical occlusion of the AChA was performed intentionally by Cooper to treat Parkinson's disease, there is no justification for intentionally occluding the AChA in contemporary aneurysm surgery short of a situation where it would be needed as a true life-saving measure. The potential for severe hemiparesis, hemisensory loss, and hemianopsia should reinforce the need for meticulous preservation of the choroidal artery and its fine branches during aneurysm clipping (**Table 4.2**).

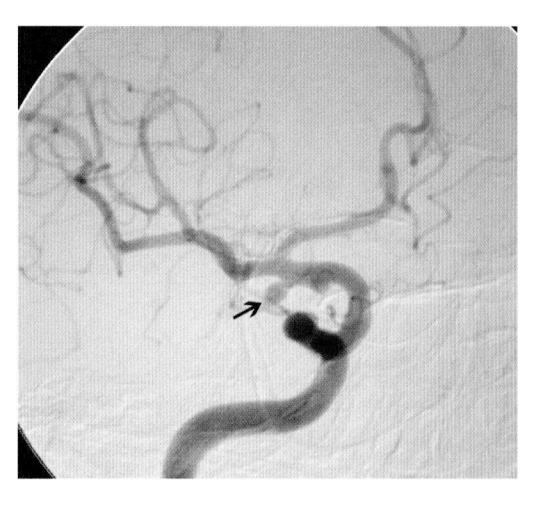

Fig. 4.9   Anteroposterior right internal carotid arteriogram demonstrates a small AChA aneurysm (*arrow*), which is treated in (VIDEO 19).

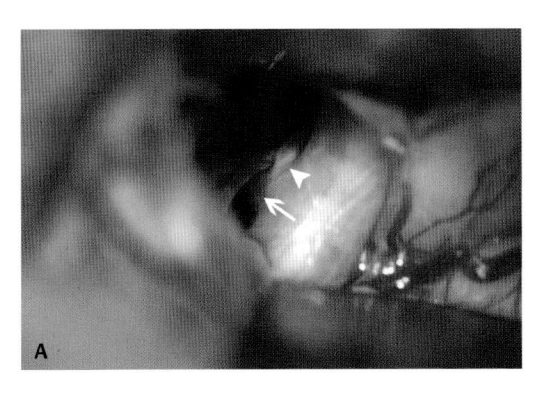

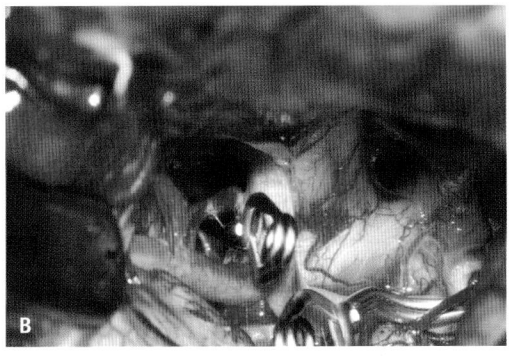

Fig. 4.10 **(A)** A tiny aneurysm (*arrow*) arising at the origin of the AChA (*arrowhead*) in a patient with multiple other aneurysms being treated at the same setting. **(B)** The aneurysm has been repaired with a clip.

Table 4.2 ■ **Anterior Choroidal Artery Aneurysm Pearls and Pitfalls**

Identify and protect the origin of the PCommA; do not mistake these for PCommA aneurysms.

Identify the origin of the AChA and free the AChA and any fine branches from the aneurysm neck as needed.

Beware of multiple or duplicated AChAs. Having identified and dissected a single AChA does not preclude the presence of a second artery hiding behind the aneurysm.

Occlusion of the PCommA can result in a PCA infarct with anterior thalmoperforating injury as well.

Occlusion of the AChA can result in contralateral hemiparesis, hemisensory loss, and hemianopsia.

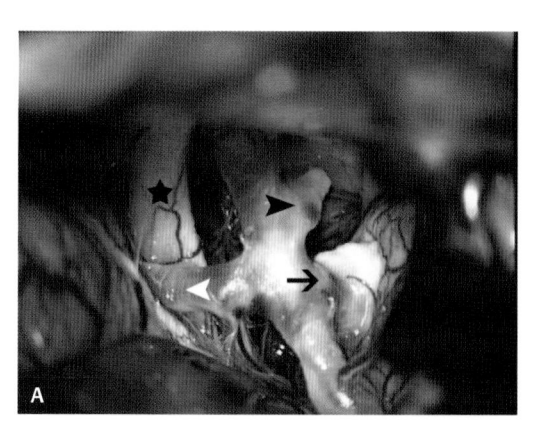

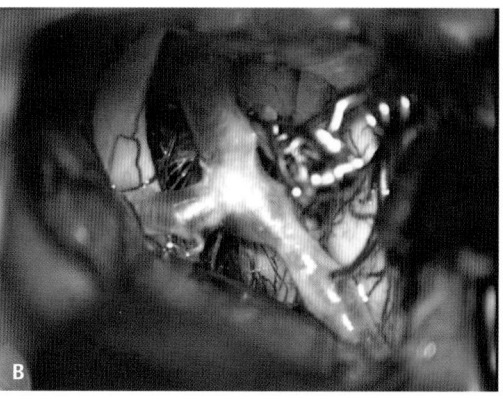

Fig. 4.11 **(A)** Left-sided posteriorly directed carotid bifurcation aneurysm (*arrow*) and anterior choroidal aneurysm (*black arrowhead*) have been exposed. The optic nerve (*star*) and the A1 segment of the anterior cerebral artery (*white arrowhead*) are also seen. **(B)** The aneurysms have been clipped.

◼ Ventral Supraclinoid Aneurysms— Dissecting Aneurysms of the ICA

Over the past decade, there has been an increasing recognition of a unique subset of aneurysms involving the ventral aspect of the supraclinoid ICA. These lesions typically present with SAH, often severe, and are usually small when first identified. They are not associated with a branching point or perforating vessel and most commonly represent dissecting aneurysms of the ICA rather than traditional saccular lesions. Angiographically, there will often be some local irregularity of the ICA, either immediately proximal or distal to the aneurysm, and this finding is often mistaken for local vasospasm. In fact, this is an important clue to the local injury to the arterial wall, reflecting the true underlying pathological process in these cases.

In the unruptured setting, we have typically been able to clip aneurysms of the ventral supraclinoid segment in straightforward fashion as one would any saccular aneurysm ⏩ VIDEO 21 . However, in the face of a recent hemorrhage, we have found these lesions to be extremely friable, often rupturing intraoperatively during gentle dissection of the aneurysm neck. In addition, we have found these lesions to be highly dynamic and unstable, often enlarging dramatically on angiographic examination from one day to the next. In addition, what appears to be a well-clipped aneurysm can quickly enlarge and rebleed over just a matter of days. Given their proximal location on the ICA, it can be difficult to achieve proximal control quickly if one has not planned appropriately in advance. Therefore, when addressing these lesions surgically, we preserve the superficial temporal artery (STA) during the opening and consider exposing the cervical ICA to offer proximal control.

Overall, we have had experience with roughly 30 ruptured, dissecting aneurysms of the ventral supraclinoid ICA. When faced with this lesion, treatment options include surgical exploration or endovascular therapy, which may consist of simple coiling when the lesion appears saccular or a stent coil construct when the aneurysm is more fusiform in nature. When these aneurysms are large, we have performed a balloon occlusion test prior to recommending a definitive course of action. If open surgery is chosen, we have sometimes been able to primarily clip an eccentric lesion ⏩ VIDEO 22 (**Fig. 4.12**). In other cases, we have used multiple fe-

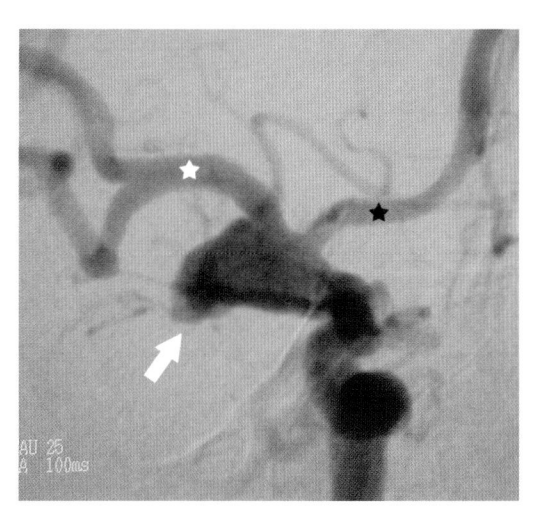

Fig. 4.12 A preoperative anteroposterior internal carotid arteriogram shows an unusual dissecting aneurysm (*arrow*) of the supraclinoid ICA that involves the proximal M1 segment (*white star*) as well. The A1 segment (*black star*) emerges from the superior aspect of the aneurysm. Treatment of this lesion is shown in ⏩ VIDEO 22 .

nestrated clips, encircling the supraclinoid ICA to reconstruct the artery (**Fig. 4.13**). Alternatively, we have at times chosen to wrap the ICA circumferentially with gauze or Gore-Tex, which is then secured with a clip (**Fig. 4.14**). Finally, we have sometimes used bypass and occlusion, a technique that will be discussed in Chapter 9, where a video of a dissecting supraclinoid ICA aneurysm treated in this fashion is presented (**Table 4.3**).

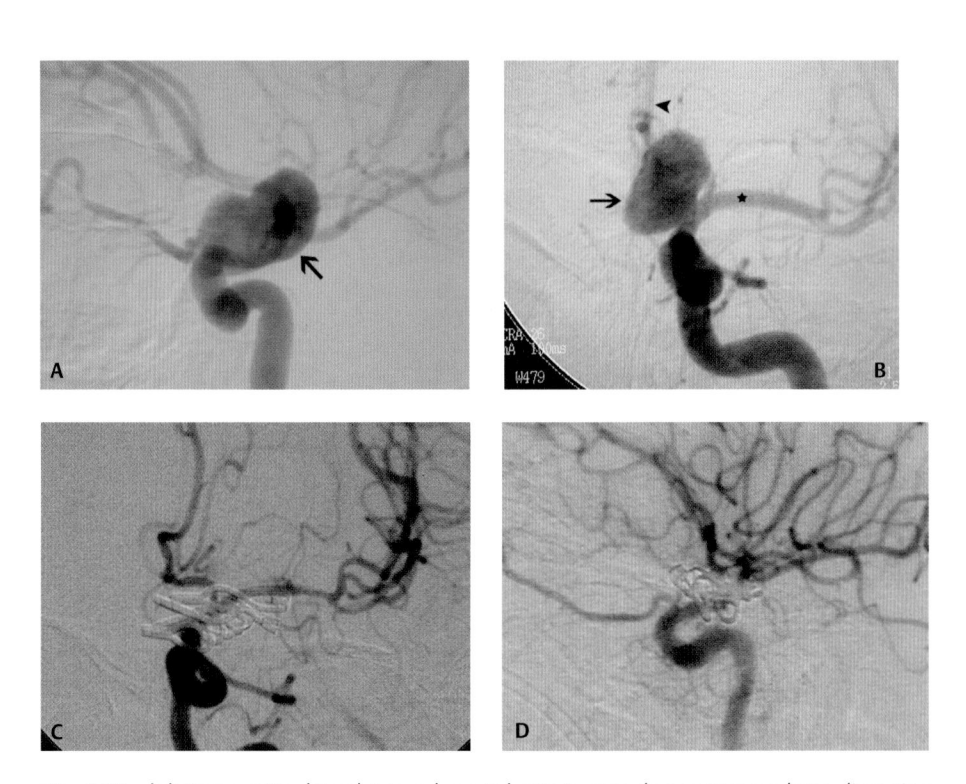

Fig. 4.13   **(A)** Preoperative lateral internal carotid arteriogram demonstrates a large dissecting aneurysm (*arrow*) of the supraclinoid ICA. **(B)** A corresponding anteroposterior angiogram demonstrates the aneurysm (*arrow*) as well the anterior cerebral (*arrowhead*) and middle cerebral (*star*) vessels. **(C)** Postoperative AP angiogram demonstrates reconstruction of the supraclinoid ICA using multiple fenestrated clips. **(D)** Corresponding lateral arteriographic image.

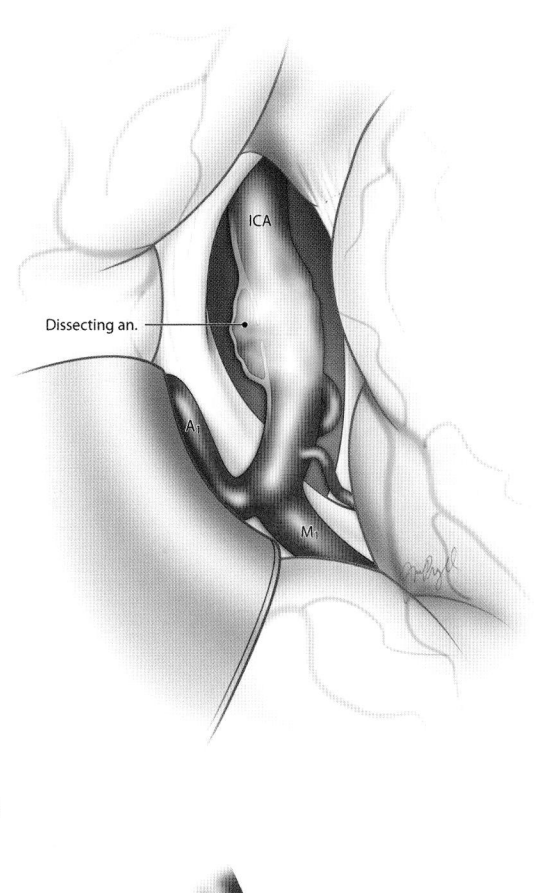

A

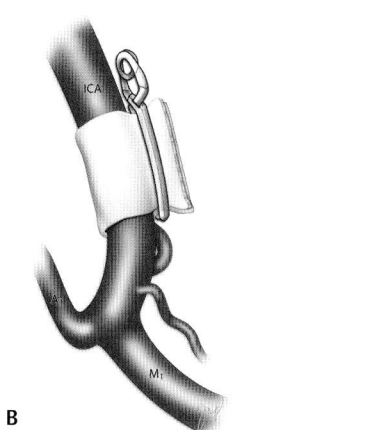

B

Fig. 4.14 Artist's illustration of a dissecting aneurysm of the ventral supraclinoid ICA **(A)** treated with circumferential wrap-clip reconstruction **(B)**.

Table 4.3 ▪ **Ventral Supraclinoid ICA Aneurysm Pearls and Pitfalls**

Preserve STA for possible bypass.

Consider exposure of cervical ICA.

Consider preoperative balloon occlusion test for larger, ruptured lesions.

Prepare distal supraclinoid ICA for temporary clipping to trap the lesion temporarily if necessary.

Beware of friability of these lesions, with high propensity for intraoperative rupture.

Beware of dynamic nature of these lesions, as angiographic appearance can change dramatically over days.

Beware of potential instability of apparently good clip reconstruction, mandating early follow-up angiographic imaging

If ICA occlusion becomes necessary, attempt to apply clip below the PCommA if possible to preserve collaterals and protect the AChA.

Severe rupture necessitating ICA occlusion can result in ischemic injury.

5 Aneurysms of the Carotid Bifurcation

Aneurysms arising at the bifurcation of the internal carotid artery (ICA) are common and can be challenging because of the frequent small perforating vessels that can be adherent to, or hidden by, these lesions. Both the recurrent artery of Heubner as well as A1 and M1 perforators will often cross these aneurysms and can be densely stuck to the aneurysm's neck or dome.

Proper exposure of these lesions requires visualization of the proximal A1 and M1 segments, and the amount of opening of the Sylvian fissure should be guided by the size and orientation of the aneurysm in these cases. As a rule, the proximal aspect of the fissure is opened sharply to reach the ICA bifurcation. This will enable visualization of the aneurysm neck. We have found it important to open the fissure further in most cases, exposing at least some length of the M1 segment (**Fig. 5.1**). In general, we prefer to dissect these aneurysms completely out of their beds, reflecting them forward to see all perforators, and then applying a permanent clip to the neck (**Fig. 5.2**). This may require a small amount of subpial resection of the deep frontal lobe, which has not carried any clinical consequence in our experience. This technique is illustrated in several videos in this collection 🔄 VIDEO 23 🔄 VIDEO 24 🔄 VIDEO 25 (**Fig. 5.3**). Once mobilized, these aneurysms can usually be clipped in straightforward fashion (**Fig. 5.4**).

ICA bifurcation aneurysms can point anteriorly, superiorly, or posteriorly. Those directed either anteriorly or superiorly are more straightforward from a surgical perspective, as they are more readily exposed through a standard pterional craniotomy 🔄 VIDEO 26 (**Fig. 5.5**). Posteriorly directed lesions point away from the surgeon and can be more difficult to expose. The surgeon must carefully identify, dissect, and separate the perforators running along the ICA bifurcation to expose the aneurysm neck (**Fig. 5.6**). These lesions can then be treated either by applying a clip over the top of the bifurcation (most common) or by working along the lateral aspect of the distal ICA above the anterior choroidal artery (AChA). In the latter instance, the surgeon must be careful not to injure the AChA. When clipping a carotid bifurcation aneurysm, it is important to avoiding placing the clip too low on the parent artery, potentially stenosing the A1 or M1 segments.

In the setting of a subarachnoid hemorrhage (SAH), establishing proximal control for an ICA bifurcation aneurysm requires access to the proximal supraclinoid ICA as well as the A1 segment. Assuming the presence of a patent anterior communicating artery (AComfA) as well as normal bilateral A1 segments, placing a temporary clip on the supraclinoid ICA may only minimally decrease the bleeding from an ICA bifurcation aneurysm that ruptures in the operating room. It should also be noted that when a carotid bifurcation aneurysm bleeds, it can occasionally result in a large hematoma involving the overlying frontal lobe. This hematoma can rupture directly into the ventricle with only minimal associated SAH. In these cases, it is important to recognize the true source of the bleeding as a ruptured ICA bifurcation aneurysm (**Table 5.1**).

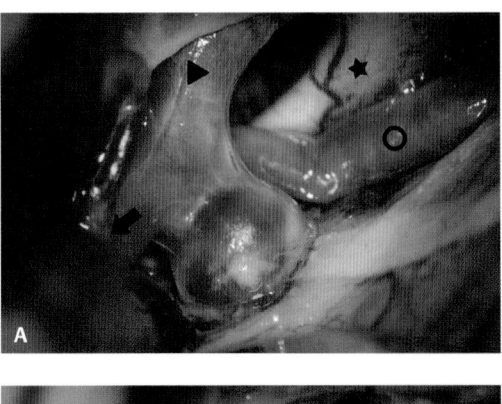

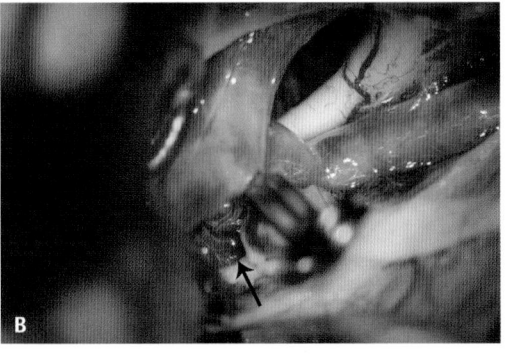

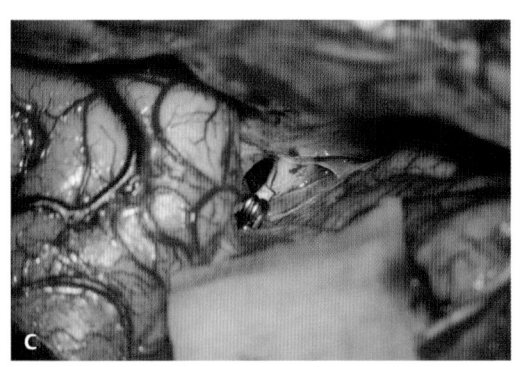

Fig. 5.1 **(A)** A small ventrally and superiorly directed aneurysm of the ICA bifurcation is exposed. Note its relationship to the supraclinoid ICA (*arrowhead*), the M1 segment (*arrow*), the A1 segment (*circle*), and the optic nerve (*star*). **(B)** The aneurysm has been clipped, and several perforators (*arrow*) are now visible behind the aneurysm. **(C)** The overall exposure and amount of opening of the Sylvian fissure are shown at the conclusion of the procedure.

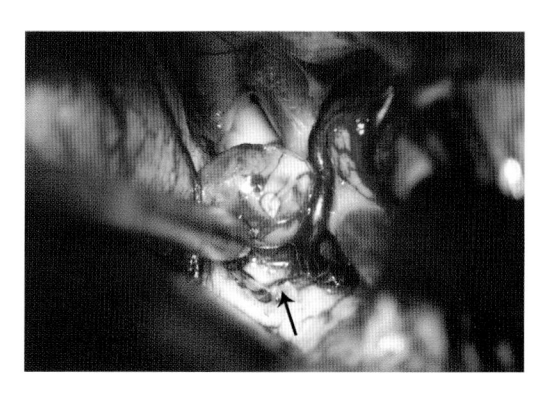

Fig. 5.2 A superiorly directed carotid bifurcation aneurysm has been reflected out of its bed (*arrow*), leaving a subfrontal vein undisturbed along the ventral aspect of the aneurysm.

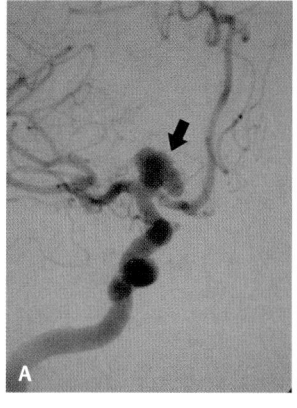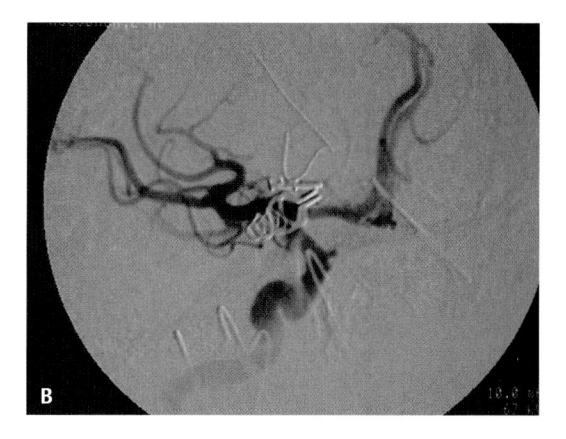

Fig. 5.3 **(A)** A complicated large and partially thrombosed carotid bifurcation aneurysm (*arrow*) is shown on a preoperative anteroposterior carotid arteriogram. **(B)** The aneurysm has been reconstructed with multiple clips on the intraoperative arteriogram. This case is shown in 🔁 VIDEO 24).

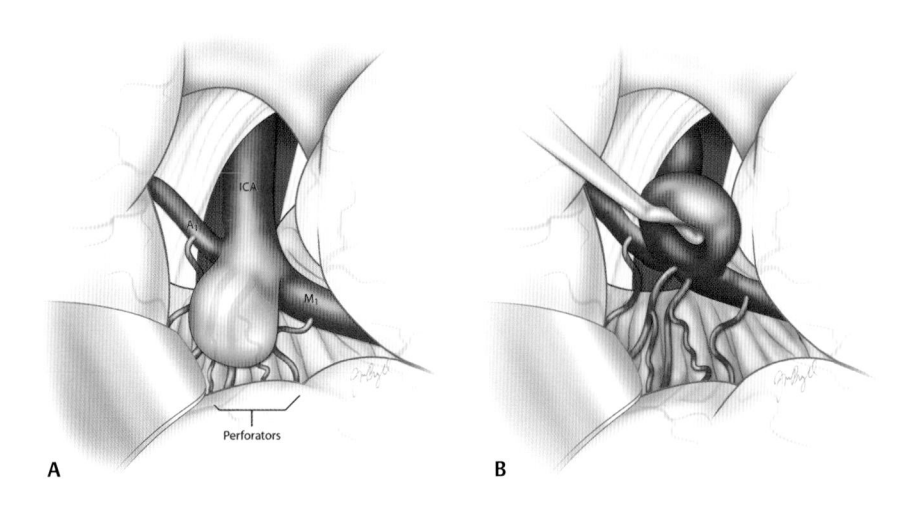

Fig. 5.4 **(A)** Artist's illustration demonstrates a wide-necked carotid bifurcation aneurysm that hides multiple perforating arteries. **(B)** The aneurysm has been fully mobilized and re-flected forward out of its bed to enable dissection and visualization of the perforating vessels behind the aneurysm prior to safe clip application.

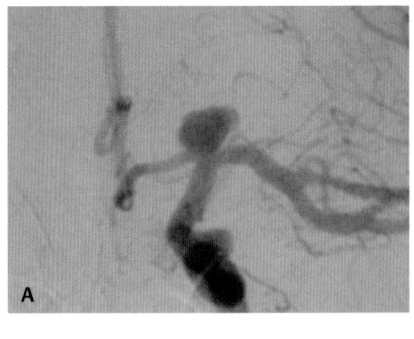
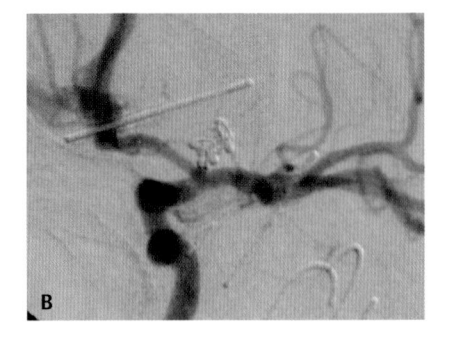

Fig. 5.5 **(A)** Preoperative anteroposterior internal carotid arteriogram demonstrates a supe-riorly directed carotid bifurcation aneurysm. **(B)** Intraoperative angiography reveals that the lesion has been repaired satisfactorily with primary neck clipping.

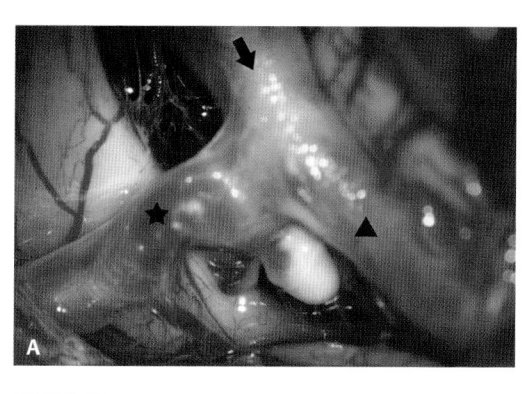

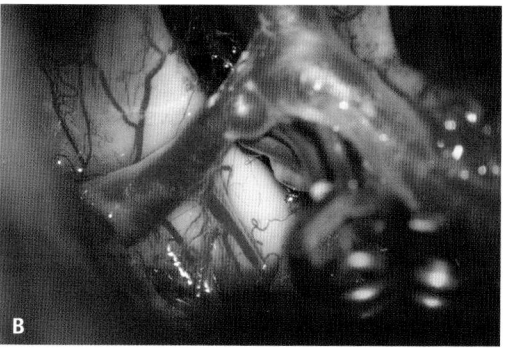

Fig. 5.6 **(A)** Two distinct posteriorly directed carotid bifurcation aneurysms are exposed along with the supraclinoid ICA (*arrow*), the M1 segment (*arrowhead*), and the A1 segment (*star*) overlying the optic nerve. The aneurysms are pointing away from the surgeon. **(B)** The lesions are clipped by working above the bifurcation, carefully preserving the associated perforators. Note the abnormal proximal A1 segment, which was subsequently wrapped with gauze.

Table 5.1 ■ **ICA Bifurcation Aneurysm Pearls and Pitfalls**

Use standard pterional craniotomy; open proximal Sylvian fissure to expose the aneurysm neck at the ICA bifurcation.

Consider fully freeing the aneurysm from its bed to properly visualize fine perforators that may be adherent to posterior aspect of dome.

Expose proximal aspect of M1 and A1 segments.

Preserve all perforating vessels.

Posteriorly directed lesions are most dangerous and difficult.

Watch the clip as it closes to avoid coming too low on the bifurcation, narrowing the A1 or less commonly the M1 segments.

Prepare distal supraclinoid ICA as well as ipsilateral A1 for temporary clipping in setting of recent rupture.

Occlusion of a deep perforator can result in contralateral hemiparesis.

6 Aneurysms of the Middle Cerebral Artery

■ M1 Segment Aneurysms

Most M1 segment aneurysms are small lesions associated with the origin of the anterior temporal artery. Although some can be coiled, many incorporate the origin of the anterior temporal itself and are best treated surgically (**Figs. 6.1, 6.2**). When the aneurysm is unruptured, we almost always open the lateral aspect of the Sylvian fissure, working from lateral to medial to follow the M2 branches back to the bifurcation and then back along the M1 trunk to the aneurysm. Over time, one develops a sense of where to begin the fissure dissection to come down directly on the aneurysm. In the setting of a ruptured M1 lesion, we will usually expose the supraclinoid internal carotid artery (ICA) proximally and then open the fissure from

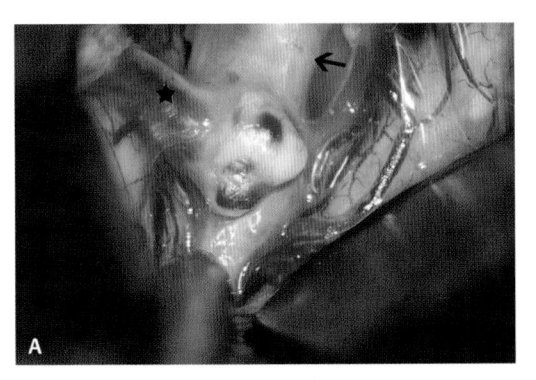

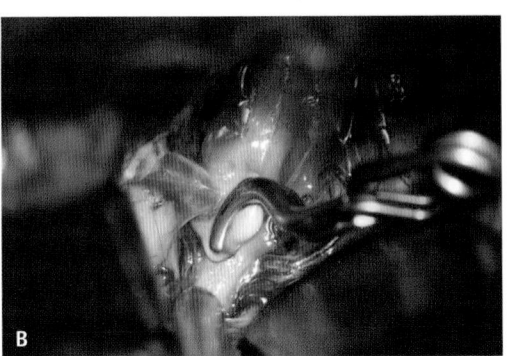

Fig. 6.1 **(A)** A small irregular aneurysm arising at the origin of the anterior temporal artery (*star*) has been exposed along with the proximal M1 segment (*arrow*) through a limited opening of the Sylvian fissure. **(B)** The lesion has been clipped.

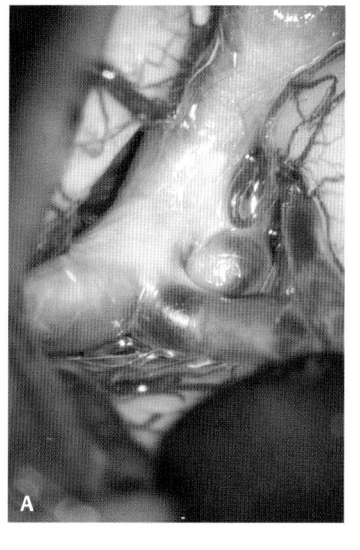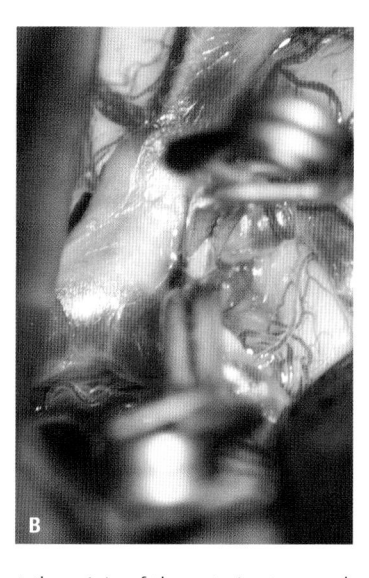

Fig. 6.2 **(A)** A small aneurysm arising at the origin of the anterior temporal artery and incorporating the artery into its base has been exposed. Note how the aneurysm is nestled between the anterior temporal artery origin and the middle cerebral bifurcation. **(B)** The aneurysm was repaired with multiple clips.

medial to lateral to achieve early proximal control. As a rule, we avoid sacrificing bridging Sylvian veins, but if the fissure cannot be opened adequately without sacrificing a tributary, it is usually well tolerated.

We have included several videos illustrating the clipping of M1 aneurysms (VIDEO 27) (VIDEO 28). Some form of intraoperative angiography is helpful to be sure that the anterior temporal artery itself has not been compromised by the clip.

Rarely, an aneurysm will arise at the origin of a lenticulostriate artery. The fine perforator will often be adherent to the aneurysm dome, and we have found these lesions best treated with very fine clips applied parallel to the M1 trunk coming across the aneurysm neck and falling just short of the lenticulostriate origin (**Fig. 6.3**). If necessary, a small amount of aneurysm can be left to preserve flow into the perforating branch and then wrapped with gauze or Gore-Tex.

Finally, we have encountered a subset of M1 aneurysms that are true fusiform lesions, which may represent dissections of the vessel (**Fig. 6.4**) (VIDEO 29). In some cases, we have been able to primarily reconstruct these lesions with a clip that gathers the saccular component, effectively reconstructing the M1 trunk. In other cases, we have used circumferential wrapping with Gore-Tex or gauze held in place with clips. In the largest of such lesions, particularly when the entire circumference of the vessel is clearly involved, distal revascularization with either proximal or distal occlusion has been an effective strategy (**Fig. 6.5**) (**Table 6.1**).

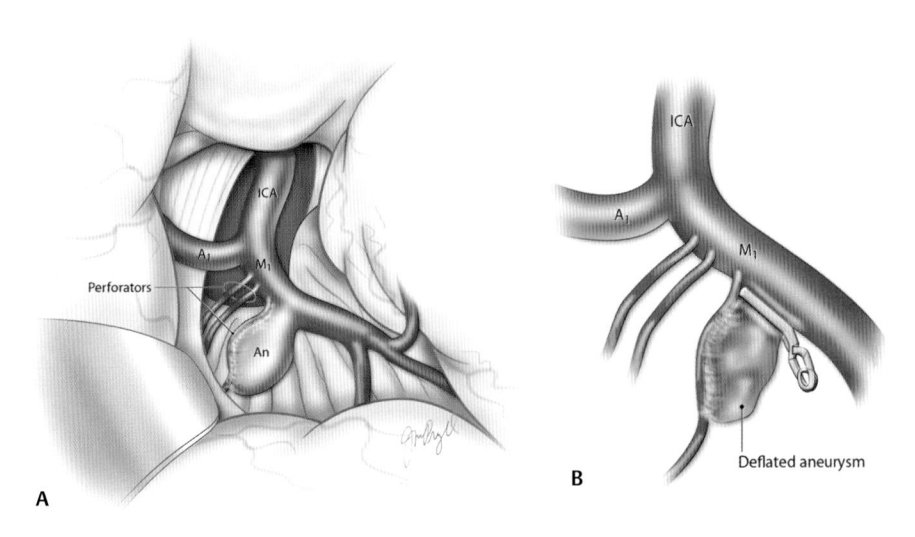

Fig. 6.3 **(A)** Artist's illustration demonstrating an aneurysm arising on the M1 segment of the middle cerebral artery with a stubbornly adherent perforating artery that cannot be safely dissected from the aneurysm neck. **(B)** The lesion has been treated by bringing a clip in parallel to the M1 segment with the tips falling just short of the perforator origin.

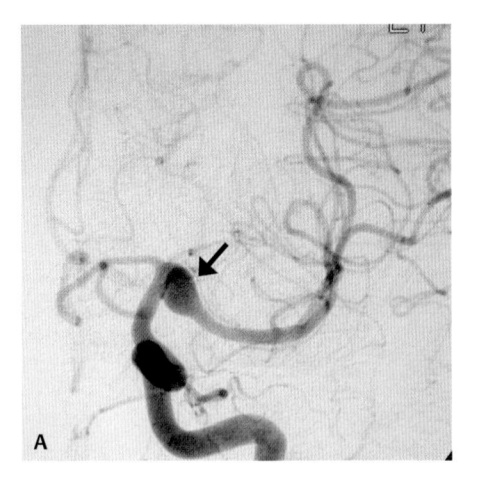

Fig. 6.4 **(A)** A fusiform M1 segment aneurysm is shown on an anteroposterior internal carotid arteriogram.

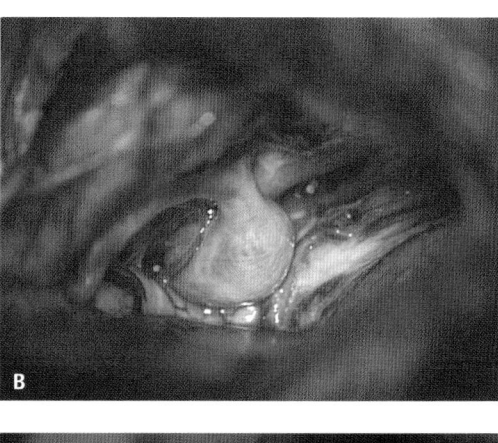

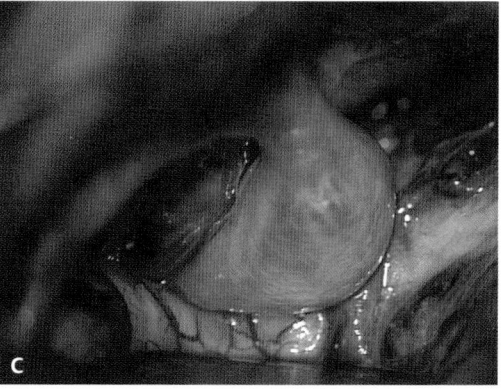

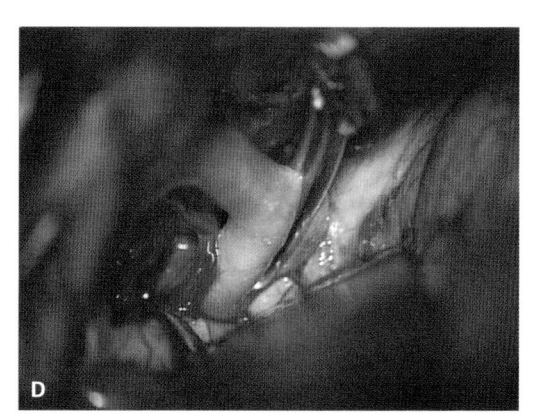

Fig. 6.4 *(Continued)*   **(B)** The Sylvian fissure has been opened to reveal the aneurysm as well as the distal M1 segment. **(C)** A more magnified view of the lesion. **(D)** The aneurysm has been reconstructed with a long clip and was subsequently wrapped with gauze.

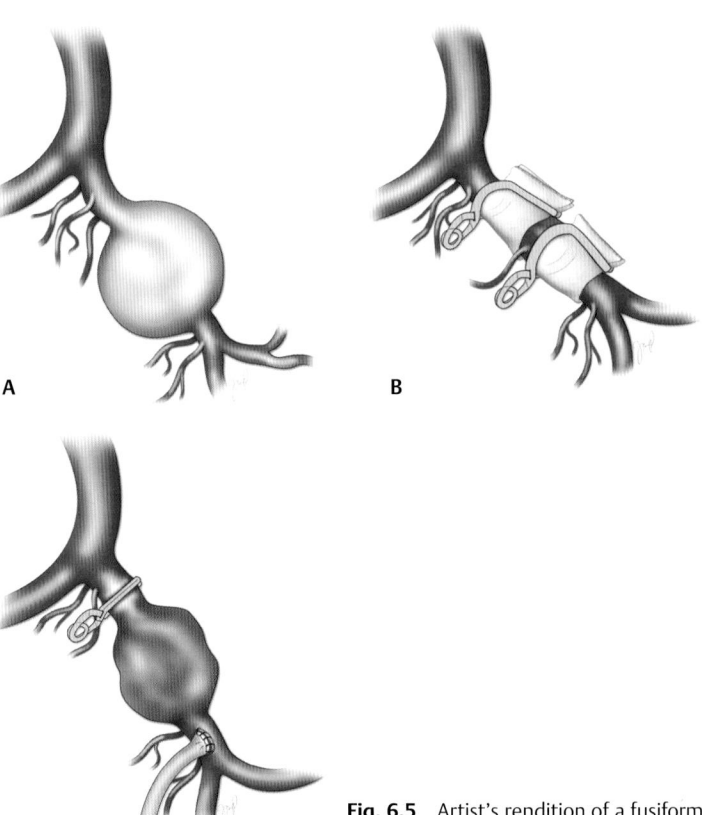

A

B

C

Fig. 6.5 Artist's rendition of a fusiform M1 segment aneurysm **(A)** demonstrating treatment options, which may include wrap/clip reconstruction **(B)** or distal revascularization with parent artery occlusion **(C)**.

Table 6.1 ■ **M1 Aneurysm Pearls and Pitfalls**

Use standard pterional craniotomy with focal opening of the Sylvian fissure.
Work from medial to lateral in the setting of SAH.
Preserve all perforating vessels off the M1.
Origin of the anterior temporal artery is often incorporated into the aneurysm neck.
Be careful to preserve all perforators, particularly when aneurysm arises at the origin of a lenticulostriate artery.
Use primary clip reconstruction, wrap/clip reinforcement, or bypass with occlusion for fusiform M1 lesions.
Occlusion of the anterior temporal artery can result in temporal lobe ischemia.
Occlusion of a lenticulostriate artery can result in a capsular infarct.

■ MCA Bifurcation Aneurysms

For most aneurysm surgeons, the middle cerebral artery (MCA) bifurcation has become the most common location of aneurysms treated surgically. This probably relates to the wide necks associated with most MCA bifurcation aneurysms, which typically incorporate one or both of the M2 branches. This provides a serious challenge for endovascular therapy, whereas surgical clip application is well suited for these lesions. Currently in our practice, we clip the vast majority of MCA aneurysms.

In the author's opinion, the emerging trend of using complex endovascular constructs such as "Y" stenting to treat these lesions is difficult to understand when a competent surgeon is available. These endovascular techniques carry significantly higher complication rates than those offered by an experienced neurovascular surgeon, and the durability of stent coil constructs in the setting of a wide-necked aneurysm cannot match that associated with proper neck clipping. Although the use of such constructs may have a role for aneurysms in locations where surgical results are less favorable (such as the basilar apex), it makes little sense to offer patients a procedure that carries a higher risk and has poorer results than open microsurgical clipping. Sadly, the growing enthusiasm for endovascular treatment performed outside the setting of a team approach that includes an experienced neurovascular surgeon has resulted in an increasing number of such cases being treated endovascularly, with an associated increase in the rates of early complications and complex, late recurrences.

For unruptured lesions, we generally use a limited opening of the lateral Sylvian fissure as described above (**Figs. 6.6, 6.7**). The opening can be extended proximally or distally as needed to afford full exposure of the aneurysm or to reach additional aneurysms at the same setting (**Fig. 6.8**). Many wide-necked lesions require multiple clips to reconstruct the MCA bifurcation properly. At times, the entire bifurcation is aneurysmal and the eccentric, saccular component can be clipped while the entire parent artery is wrapped with gauze or Gore-Tex that can be secured

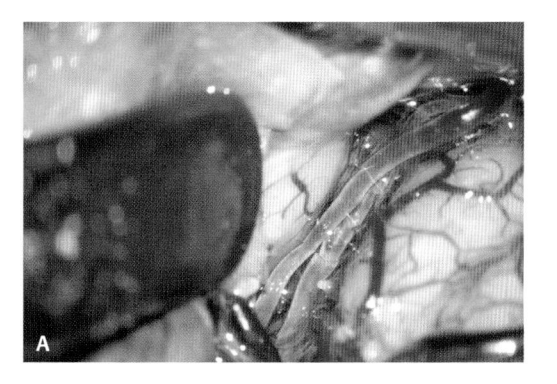

Fig. 6.6   (A) Series of photomicrographs illustrating opening of the superficial Sylvian fissure. *(Continued on page 64)*

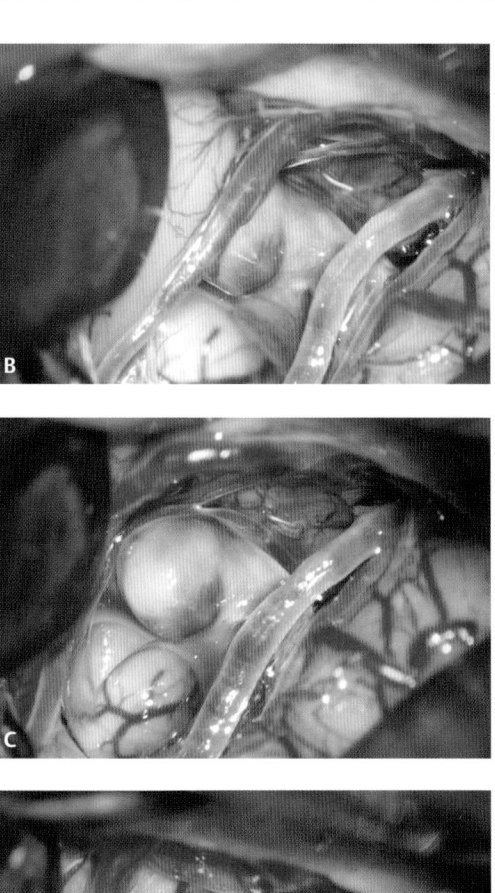

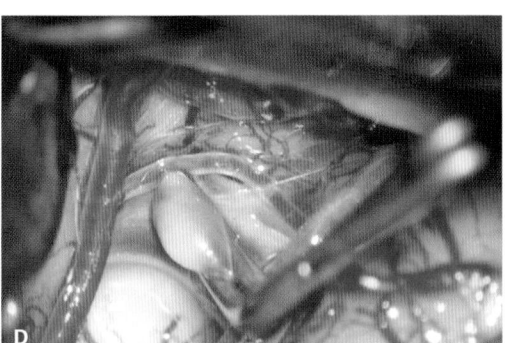

Fig. 6.6 *(Continued)* **(B)** A first glimpse of a middle cerebral artery bifurcation aneurysm is offered. **(C)** The aneurysm has been dissected. **(D)** A clip has been applied.

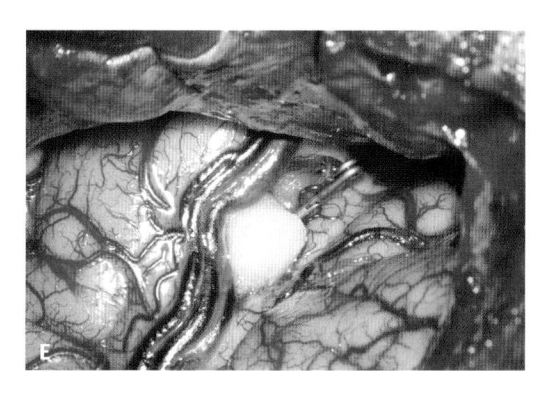

Fig. 6.6 *(Continued)*   **(E)** The limited extent of the Sylvian opening can be seen in the final image.

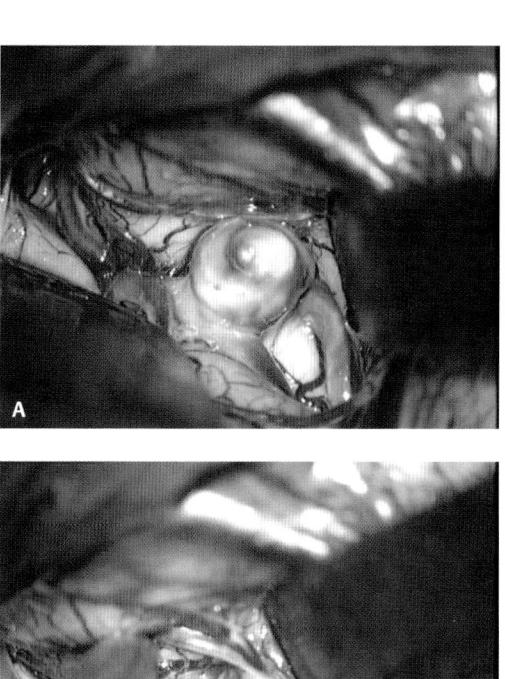

Fig. 6.7   **(A)** A classic example of a lateral Sylvian opening to expose a small MCA aneurysm. **(B)** The dome is reflected with a dissector to properly expose the hidden origin of one of the M2 branches. *(Continued on page 66)*

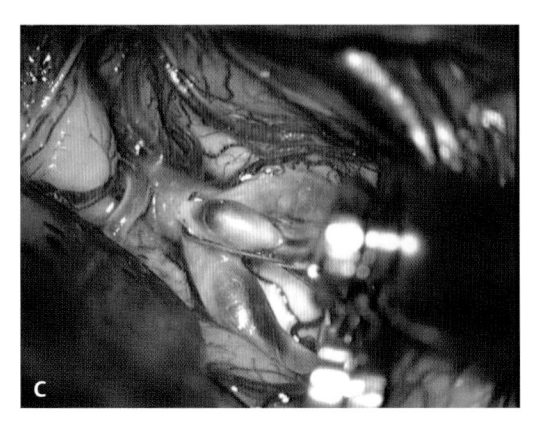

Fig. 6.7 *(Continued)*   **(C)** The lesion has been clipped.

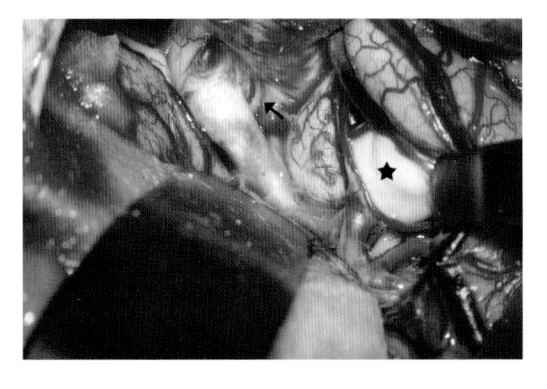

Fig. 6.8   Full opening of the Sylvian fissure is shown to visualize a posteriorly directed para-clinoid aneurysm (*arrow*) as well as a partially calcified middle cerebral bifurcation aneurysm (*star*). Note the white atheromatous wall of the MCA aneurysm.

circumferentially around the vessel (**Fig. 6.9**). In general, it is better to leave some "fullness" at the MCA bifurcation than to stenose the origins of one or both M2 branches, risking a serious ischemic injury.

We have included multiple MCA aneurysm examples in this series to highlight the variety of nuances and techniques that we have found useful in clipping these lesions 👁 VIDEO 30) 👁 VIDEO 31) 👁 VIDEO 32) 👁 VIDEO 33) 👁 VIDEO 34) 👁 VIDEO 35). Younger surgeons should focus on becoming adept at opening the Sylvian fissure using sharp microsurgical dissection while avoiding pial transgression (**Fig. 6.10**). This represents an excellent microsurgical exercise as well as the cornerstone of surgery for anterior circulation aneurysms and MCA aneurysms, in

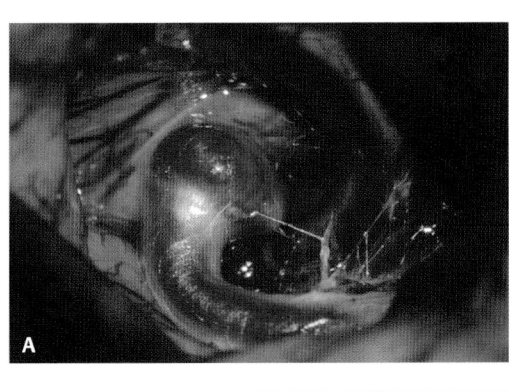

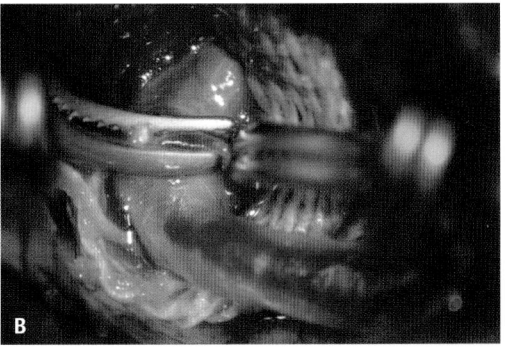

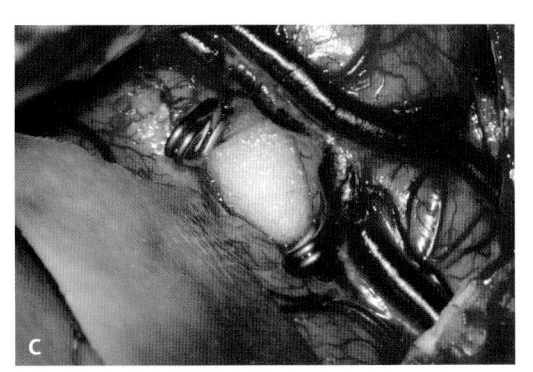

Fig. 6.9 **(A)** A small and thin-walled MCA bifurcation aneurysm in a 19-year-old woman has been exposed. **(B)** Gauze has been introduced in preparation for wrapping of the bulbous bifurcation after clip occlusion of the aneurysm itself. **(C)** The limited Sylvian opening is highlighted.

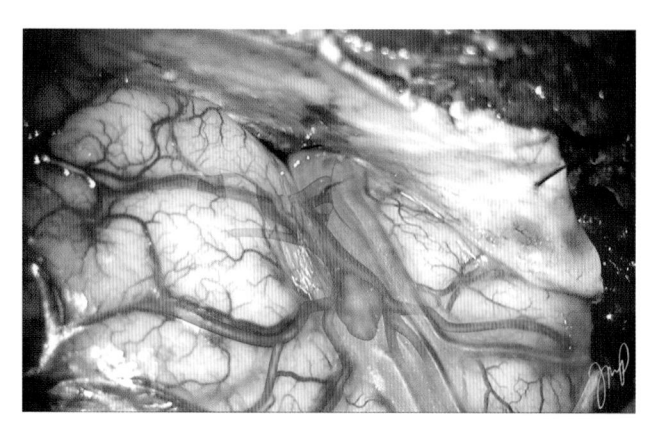

Fig. 6.10   Artist's operative photographic overlay illustrating the relationship of a typical MCA aneurysm to the overlying Sylvian fissure.

particular. For larger aneurysms, it may be helpful to free the dome fully from its bed, enabling precise clip reconstruction. In select cases, multiple clips can be used to reconstruct a complex aneurysm, or fenestrated clips may be useful, allowing the surgeon to leave a densely adherent branch attached to the aneurysm dome (**Figs. 6.11, 6.12**). When the M1 segment is short, it may be easier to open the fissure from medial to lateral. In such cases, one should be careful to preserve every small vessel running near the aneurysm, as medial lenticulostriate vessels irrigating the internal capsule can be injured when treating a bifurcation aneurysm arising on a short M1 segment.

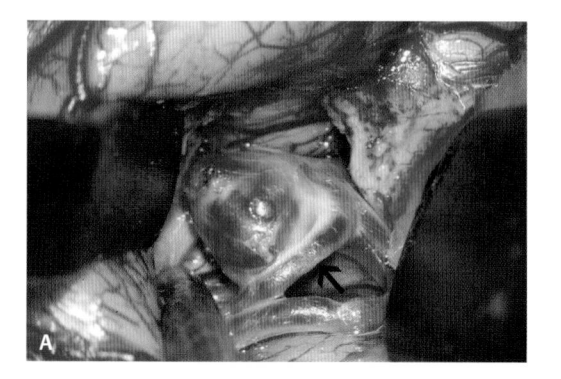

Fig. 6.11   **(A)** An M2 branch (*arrow*) is extremely adherent to the middle cerebral bifurcation aneurysm.

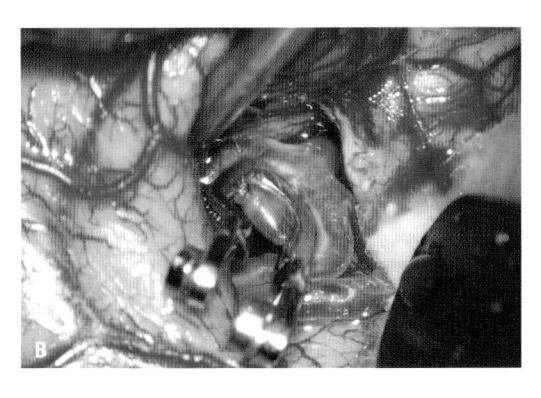

Fig. 6.11 *(Continued)*   **(B)** The lesion has been treated with multiple clips that leave the adherent branch attached to the aneurysm.

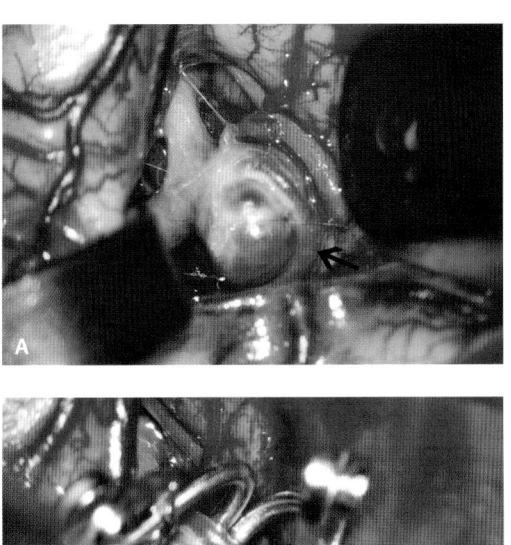

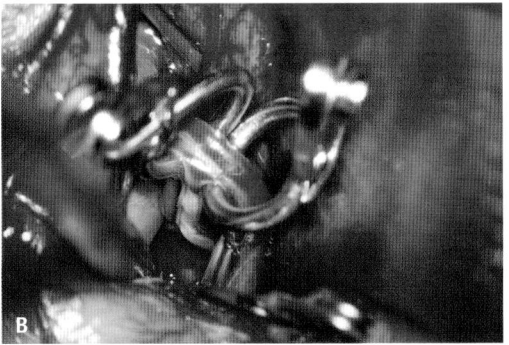

Fig. 6.12   **(A)** A small branch *(arrow)* is seen arising from the base of this middle cerebral aneurysm. The branch runs along and is tightly adherent to the dome. **(B)** The lesion is therefore treated with fenestrated clips that leave the branch open in their fenestrations while occluding the aneurysm.

On occasion, middle cerebral aneurysms can present with a large temporal lobe hematoma, potentially resulting in a life-threatening cerebral herniation syndrome. As described in Chapter 4, we bring these patients to the operating room without a formal preoperative diagnostic angiogram, perform a generous craniotomy, open the dura, and then perform an intraoperative angiogram to map the vascular anatomy (**Fig. 6.13**). The hematoma can then be evacuated, and the aneurysm can be treated, although we prefer to avoid working through the hematoma cavity to reach the aneurysm if at all possible. When treating smaller ruptured aneurysms of the MCA, we prefer to expose the M1 segment first to achieve proximal control and then dissect the aneurysm itself, often with the use of temporary clipping (**Fig. 6.14**).

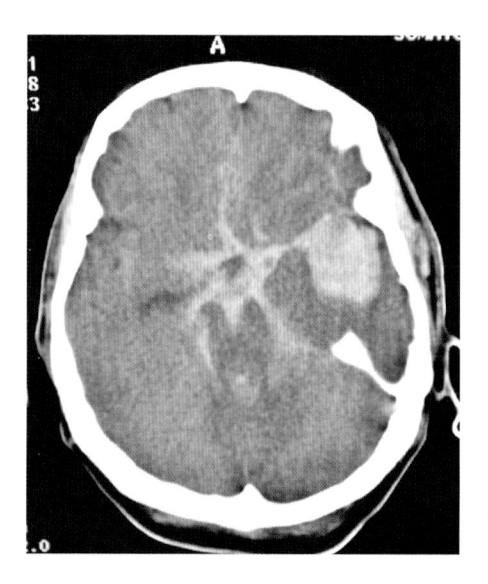

Fig. 6.13   An axial CT scan demonstrates a large Sylvian hematoma resulting from the rupture of a giant MCA aneurysm, resulting in an acute herniation syndrome.

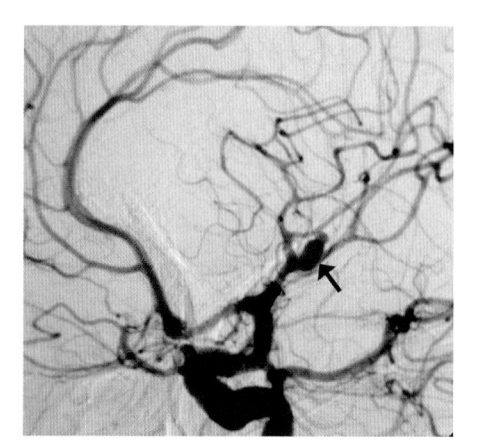

Fig. 6.14   Oblique internal carotid angiography reveals a small ruptured MCA aneurysm (*arrow*) in a patient with a severe subarachnoid hemorrhage (SAH). This lesion is treated in ⏵VIDEO 35 .

Table 6.2　■　MCA Bifurcation Aneurysm Pearls and Pitfalls

Standard pterional craniotomy with limited lateral opening of the Sylvian fissure is satisfactory for most unruptured lesions.

When ruptured, expose the M1 segment before the aneurysm is dissected.

Preserve all perforating vessels.

Be careful when treating MCA bifurcation aneurysm with short M1 segment, as critical lenticulostriates can run past aneurysm.

M2 branches are typically incorporated into the aneurysm base, necessitating creative clip constructs.

It is often better to leave the MCA bifurcation slightly bulbous than to stenose the origin of the M2 vessels.

Beware of following a hematoma cavity down to a ruptured aneurysm without first achieving proximal control and a good understanding of the critical anatomy at the neck of the aneurysm.

Bypass is useful in giant lesions.

Injury to Sylvian veins can result in venous ischemia.

Occlusion of a lenticulostriate can result in a capsular infarct.

Occlusion of an M2 branch can result in hemispheric ischemia:
Contralateral hemparesis
Hemisensory loss
Dysphasia

The MCA bifurcation is one of the most common locations to encounter a giant aneurysm. The management of giant aneurysms is detailed in Chapter 9. In these cases, bypass has become an important part of our treatment algorithm, with primary clip reconstruction or aneurysmorrhaphy representing alternative options (**Table 6.2**).

■ Distal MCA Aneurysms

Distal MCA aneurysms most often occur on M2 branches and can be approached just as one would an MCA bifurcation aneurysm. The Sylvian fissure is opened more laterally to offer full exposure of the M2 branches (**Fig. 6.15**). Careful dissection will allow the surgeon to continue following the fissure out quite laterally, exposing M3 and even M4 branches as needed. In some cases, a localizing intraoperative angiogram, or possibly intraoperative neuronavigation, can be very helpful to locate the lesion.

More peripheral aneurysms may represent dissections or may be mycotic in origin and should be treated at centers with significant experience in vascular re-

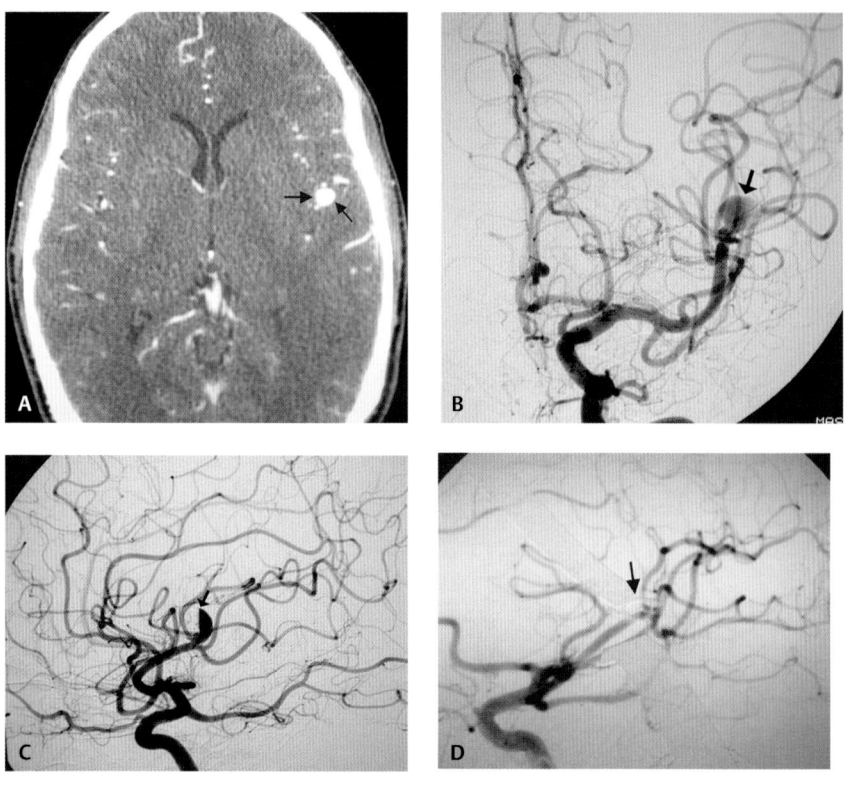

Fig. 6.15 **(A)** This patient presented with a minor SAH from a peripherally situated middle cerebral aneurysm (*arrow*), which can be seen on the contrast-enhanced axial CT scan. **(B)** Anteroposterior internal carotid arteriogram shows the peripheral aneurysm (*arrow*). **(C)** Note the partial thrombosis within the aneurysm (*arrow*), as shown on the lateral arteriogram. **(D)** The lesion was treated surgically, with an intraoperative arteriogram revealing occlusion of the aneurysm (*arrow*) with sparing of the normal vessels. (*Images reprinted with permission from the Journal of Neurosurgery.*)

construction. Primary clip reconstruction may not be feasible in these situations, and excision with end-to-end reconstruction or distal bypass with occlusion may become necessary. We have included a video of one such lesion, treated by preliminary external carotid–internal carotid (EC-IC) bypass followed by trapping and excision of the aneurysm ⟳ VIDEO 36).

It is worth noting that there has been a growing trend in the endovascular community to rely on simple parent artery occlusion in the treatment of peripheral aneurysms. We feel strongly that surgical exploration is warranted in the majority of such cases. This allows the surgeon to possibly reconstruct the artery primarily with clips or to consider some form of distal revascularization if an occlusion becomes necessary. In our experience, the involved arterial branch is often larger than normal in these cases, and these "end" arteries may have little or no collateral supply, further tempering our enthusiasm for simple parent artery occlusion (**Table 6.3**).

Table 6.3 ▪ **Distal MCA Aneurysm Pearls and Pitfalls**

Use standard pterional craniotomy with posterior extension as needed to reach the aneurysm.
Open lateral Sylvian fissure, carefully following M2 branches as far as necessary.
Intraoperative angiography or neuronavigation can be helpful to localize more distal lesions, as it can be difficult to find the aneurysm.
Distal branches may be small and harder to preserve with standard clipping techniques.
The distal MCA has increased incidence of mycotic and fusiform lesions, which may be friable and circumferentially involve vessel.
Open surgical exploration is preferable to endovascular parent artery occlusion in most cases to avoid ischemic injury.
Consider excision with end-to-end reanastomosis or a short jump graft in these cases.
Inability to reconstruct aneurysm, necessitating parent artery occlusion, can result in ischemic injury.

7 Aneurysms of the Basilar Artery

■ Basilar Apex Aneurysms

Basilar apex aneurysms should be treated by experienced aneurysm surgeons. Today, the majority of basilar apex aneurysms can be managed endovascularly with primary coiling or a stent-coil construct. Those aneurysms not amenable to coiling generally represent surgical challenges; they tend to have wider necks and often incorporate a large portion of the basilar apex as well as one or both P1 origins. The decision to treat a basilar apex aneurysm surgically is a serious one and should not be undertaken lightly. More so than at any other location, surgical treatment of a basilar apex aneurysm leaves no room for error. Occlusion of even the smallest perforator can result in devastating consequences to the patient. Although imperfect in terms of durability, endovascular options have generally resulted in dramatically improved neurological outcomes compared with open surgery, as most surgeons are not able to clip apex aneurysms reliably without incurring significant morbidity for their patients.

When surgery is planned, the choice of approach will depend on surgical experience, personal preference, and aneurysm orientation. Options include the subtemporal, pterional, and half-half procedures, which can be augmented by skull base dissections such as an orbitozygomatic (OZ) osteotomy. We have included several videos of basilar apex lesions because of their relative rarity, including examples of each of the above approaches ⟳ VIDEO 37) ⟳ VIDEO 38) ⟳ VIDEO 39). Adequate brain relaxation and a certain amount of intraoperative flexibility are important so that the surgeon is able to adapt to the specific anatomy encountered. Apex perforators must be preserved without exception, and temporary clipping of the distal basilar artery (BA), either below or immediately above the origins of the superior cerebellar arteries (SCAs), is an important tool to soften larger aneurysms that fill a tight working area. Note that the author has no experience with the so-called "transcavernous" approach to the basilar apex, as we have preferred to avoid opening the cavernous sinus in this setting.

In the setting of a serious subarachnoid hemorrhage (SAH), some form of cerebrospinal fluid (CSF) drainage is mandatory when approaching a basilar apex aneurysm. We generally prefer a ventricular drain, although a spinal drain is a reasonable alternative, assuming the fourth ventricle is not occluded by fresh clot. Early in our experience, when treating an unruptured BA lesion, we always used a lumbar drainage catheter. More recently, we have found that aggressive opening of the basal cisterns will generally provide adequate relaxation if one is patient at the beginning of the operation. When utilizing a true subtemporal approach, the use of a spinal drain remains an important surgical adjunct.

The Pterional Approach

The various approaches to the basilar apex carry advantages and disadvantages (**Fig. 7.1**). The main advantage of the pterional approach is its familiarity to the aneurysm surgeon. Since it is used for the treatment of almost all anterior circulation aneurysms, the aneurysm surgeon should be extremely comfortable working through this familiar trajectory. We have found that aggressive drilling of the anterior clinoid process and opening of the falciform ligament allow the surgeon to mobilize the optic nerve, increasing the working angle to the basilar apex. It is striking how even a small amount of increased working room can dramatically change the situation from an almost impossible one to a manageable challenge.

By opening the Sylvian fissure widely, the surgeon can untether the attachments of the medial temporal lobe. Mobilization of the medial temporal lobe will enable the surgeon to work past the internal carotid artery (ICA) along the course of the posterior communicating artery (PCommA) and anterior choroidal artery (AChA) to reach and open the membrane of Lilliquiest. At this point, the surgeon will have to decide the best trajectory to the basilar apex. This will depend heavily on the local vascular anatomy. Most often, the space between the ICA and third nerve will pro-

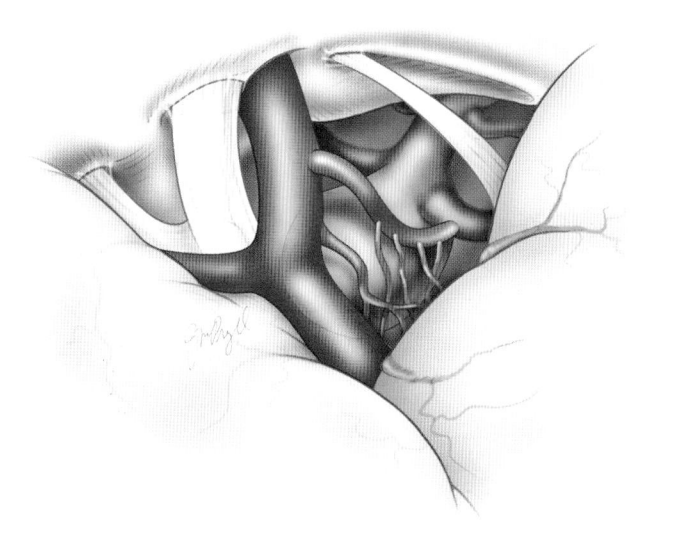

Fig. 7.1 Artist's illustration of a pterional approach to a basilar apex aneurysm. The working angle is somewhat narrow. Note how division of the posterior communicating artery (PCommA) could expand the working window in such a case.

vide the best exposure (**Figs. 7.2–7.4**). In some cases, the anatomy affords a generous working angle between the optic nerve and ICA (**Fig. 7.5**). Rarely, the surgeon can work over the top of a short supraclinoid ICA, but in such a circumstance, one must diligently protect all medial lenticulostriate perforators.

The main disadvantage of the pterional approach is the limited working angle to the basilar apex. In some cases, the exposure can be improved by dividing the PCommA judiciously between anterior thalamoperforating arteries. Because the PCommA represents an important potential source of collateral supply to the upper BA, we have avoided using this maneuver when the PCommA is large. It should be noted that low-lying aneurysms of the basilar apex will be hidden by the posterior clinoid process and can be almost impossible to treat using a pterional approach unless one is prepared to remove the posterior clinoid. In addition, the surgeon must work past several normal critical structures, and when focused intently on the deep anatomy within the interpeduncular cistern, it can be challenging to avoid their inadvertent damage. In particular, the literature bears testament to cases of carotid laceration, optic nerve injury, and third-nerve contusion during the treatment of basilar apex aneurysms.

When the M1 is short, it can be difficult to mobilize the medial temporal lobe adequately, and the anterior temporal artery can be easily stretched or even avulsed during deep retraction of the temporal pole. Finally, the pterional approach gives the surgeon a relatively anterior view of the basilar apex. For more narrow-necked lesions, this may be adequate, but when the aneurysm has a very broad base in the coronal plane, it can be difficult to fully visualize the apex perforators hidden behind the aneurysm dome. In such cases, Samson and Batjer have advocated reflecting the entire aneurysm from its bed, much as we do with ICA bifurcation aneurysms. Unfortunately, for all but the most experienced of aneurysm surgeons, the idea of reflecting a large basilar apex aneurysm out of its bed deep within the interpeduncular fossa is a daunting task with potentially devastating consequences.

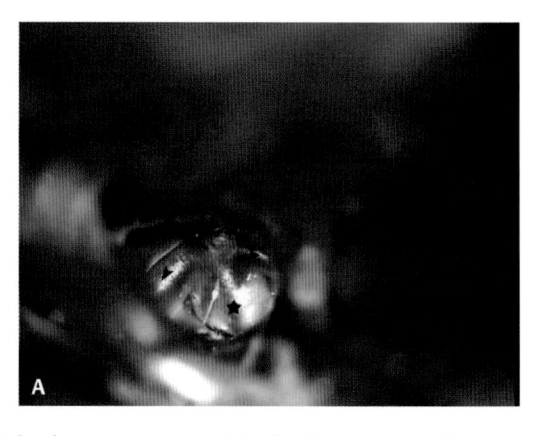

Fig. 7.2 **(A)** A basilar apex aneurysm (*star*) has been exposed through a classic pterional approach. A ventral view of the basilar apex is afforded, and both P1 segments (*arrowheads*) are nicely visualized while working between the ICA and third nerve.

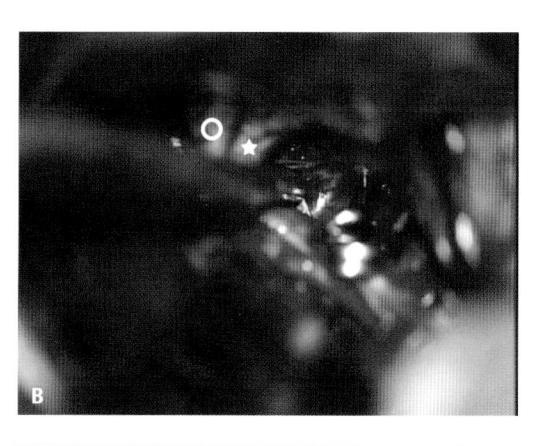

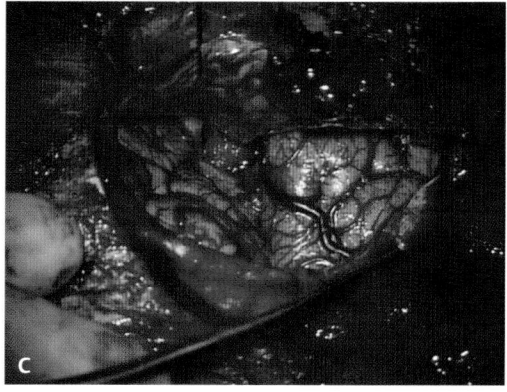

Fig. 7.2 *(Continued)*   **(B)** The aneurysm has been clipped and the ICA (*white star*) is being retracted forward toward the optic nerve (*white circle*) with the suction. **(C)** An overview photomicrograph of the pterional exposure is provided as well.

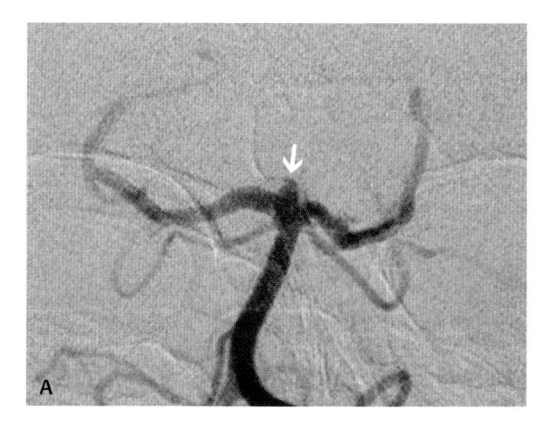

Fig. 7.3   **(A)** A small, ruptured, blisterlike aneurysm (*arrow*) of the basilar apex is visualized on a preoperative vertebral arteriogram. *(Continued on page 78)*

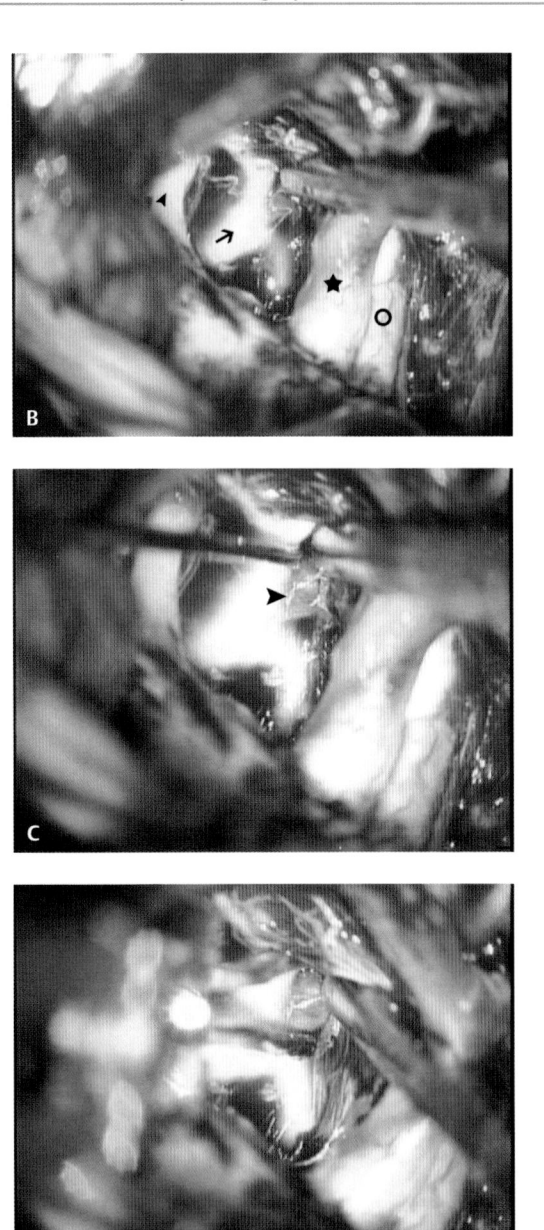

Fig. 7.3 *(Continued)*   **(B)** Through a pterional approach, the upper basilar artery (*arrow*) is exposed by working between the ICA (*star*) and the third cranial nerve (*arrowhead*). The optic nerve (*circle*) is seen in front of the carotid artery. **(C)** The neck of the aneurysm (*arrowhead*) is being dissected. **(D)** A clip is being applied across the aneurysm neck. This case is shown in ⏵VIDEO 37).

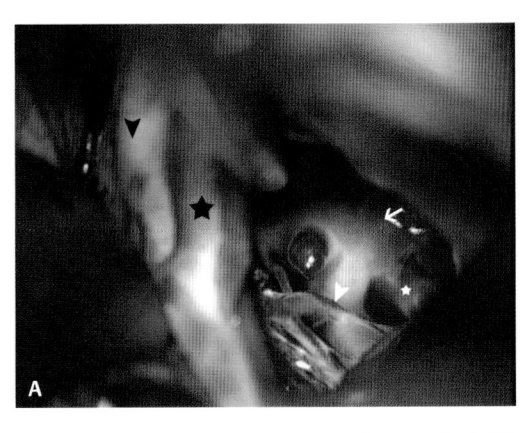

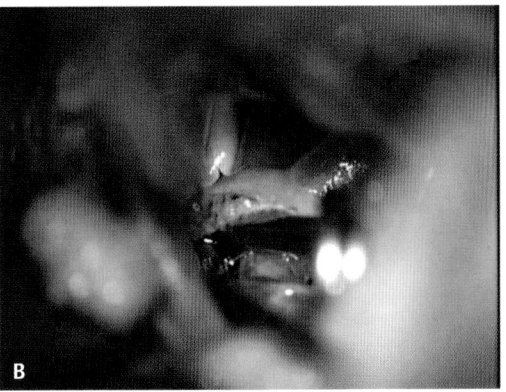

Fig. 7.4 **(A)** A small, blisterlike basilar apex aneurysm has been exposed through a pterional approach. The optic nerve (*black arrowhead*) and ICA (*black star*) are retracted gently forward with the suction to widen the working angle. The BA (*white arrow*), SCA (*white star*), and the junction between the PCommA and the P1 segment of the posterior cerebral artery (PCA) (*white arrowhead*) are all nicely visualized. **(B)** The aneurysm has been clipped and gauze wrapped around the clip construct, given the young age of the patient in this case.

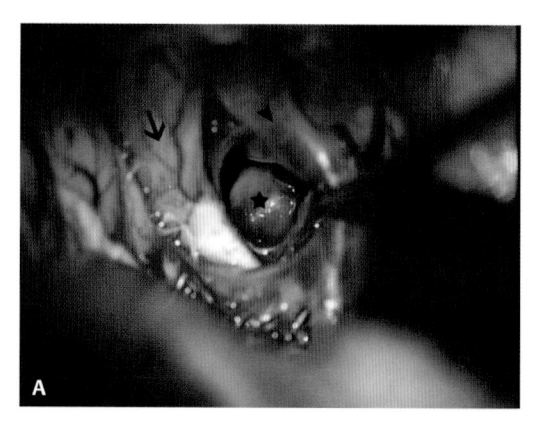

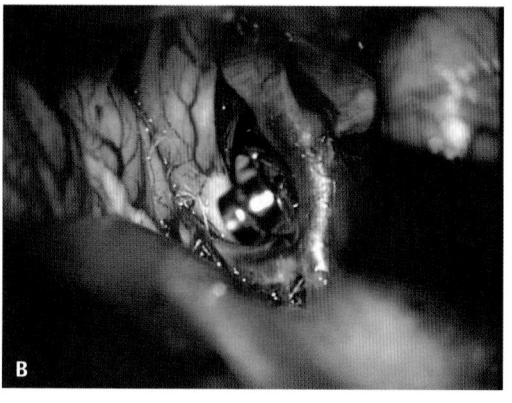

Fig. 7.5   **(A)** A basilar apex aneurysm (*star*) is exposed in this case by working between the internal carotid artery (*arrowhead*) and the optic nerve (*arrow*). **(B)** The aneurysm has been clipped.

Subtemporal

The subtemporal approach as pioneered by Drake is elegant in terms of its simplicity (**Fig. 7.6**). A small temporal craniotomy, coming down to the floor of the middle cranial fossa, is performed. Spinal or ventricular drainage is necessary to provide adequate brain relaxation. The temporal lobe is then gradually elevated using several large retractors to distribute the force of retraction over as large an area as possible (**Fig. 7.7**). Once the incisura is visualized, the tentorial edge is divided behind the insertion of the fourth cranial nerve, and a suture is used to widen the exposure. It is often surprising how much additional working space is afforded by this simple maneuver. At this point, the deeper arachnoid reflections are taken down sharply, and the PCA is identified and followed back to the basilar apex.

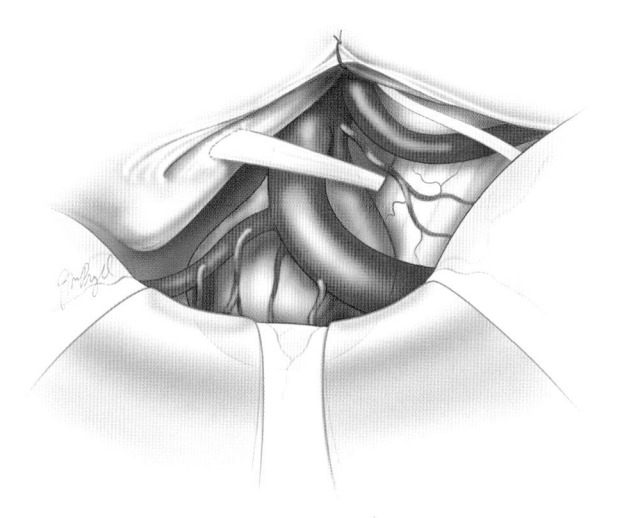

Fig. 7.6 Subtemporal exposure of a basilar apex aneurysm, depicting the access afforded to the posterior aspect of the aneurysm, where multiple perforators can be separated from the aneurysm under direct vision.

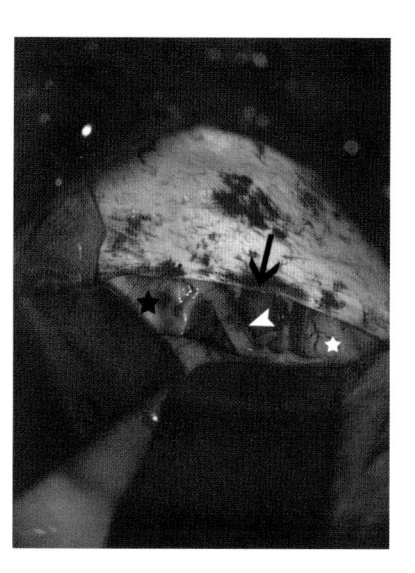

Fig. 7.7 A traditional subtemporal approach has been performed to expose the tentorial edge (*arrow*). The third cranial nerve (*arrowhead*) is seen crossing the field. The brainstem (*white star*) is visible posteriorly, and a giant basilar aneurysm (*black star*) can be seen more anteriorly.

The greatest advantage of the subtemporal approach is the excellent visualization of the basilar apex from a lateral perspective, offering the surgeon an optimal view of the anatomy behind the aneurysm dome and allowing for straightforward dissection and protection of perforators hiding behind a larger apex aneurysm. The most relevant anatomy—the posterior aspect of the neck of the aneurysm—is most easily visualized using this approach. The greatest limitations associated with the subtemporal exposure include the limited working space and the potential for inadequate visualization of the contralateral P1 and its perforators. We have found a tendency for a clip applied using the subtemporal approach to angle upward across the basilar apex, potentially leaving a dog ear above the opposite P1 origin. By being aware of this problem, we have been able to limit it. In addition, we have found that as the clip is gently closed across the basilar apex, the true anatomy of the opposite P1 often comes into view. At this point, the final dissection can be completed, and if the clip needs to be reapplied, it can now be done more precisely. Of further note, as observed by Drake, the subtemporal approach lends itself particularly well to the use of a fenestrated clip, placing the ipsilateral P1 segment in the fenestration as the blades close across the aneurysm neck (**Fig. 7.8**). Once the fenestrated clip is applied, the neck can be inspected fully. At this point, it is sometimes possible to tilt the dome forward from its bed, enabling placement of a new clip above the first and in front of the P1. The fenestrated clip can then be adjusted or even removed as necessary, particularly if it comes down low on the basilar artery.

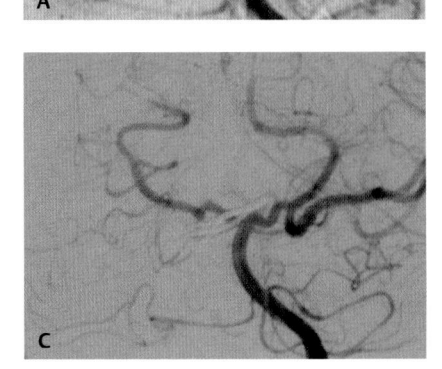

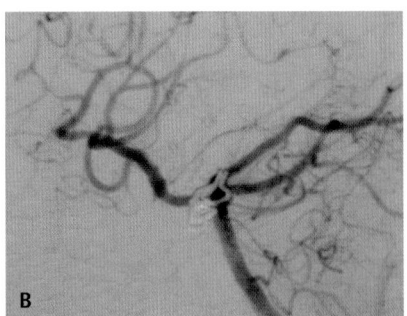

Fig. 7.8 **(A)** Preoperative AP vertebral arteriogram demonstrates a large, ruptured basilar apex aneurysm (*arrow*) which was treated using a subtemporal approach. Note the wide neck with both P1 segments (*stars*) emerging from the aneurysm base. **(B)** Postoperative lateral arteriogram demonstrates obliteration of the aneurysm using a fenestrated clip that incorporates the P1 origin. Note the large PCommA, which fills forward from the PCA on the lateral arteriographic image. **(C)** Corresponding postoperative AP arteriogram demonstrating adequate clip reconstruction of the basilar apex.

Half-half

The so-called "half half" approach represents a compromise position between the pterional and subtemporal approaches (**Fig. 7.9**). In practice, it provides an extremely robust exposure of the upper basilar artery, giving the surgeon excellent orientation and exposure of the relevant anatomy. The ICA and optic nerve are exposed as usual for a pterional approach. The PCommA and AChA are then followed posteriorly, and the tentorium can be sectioned as during a subtemporal exposure. By retracting the temporal lobe posteriorly and superiorly, the posterior fossa is exposed and the relevant anatomy revealed (**Figs. 7.10, 7.11**). The great advantage of the half-half approach is the wide exposure and the potential to treat additional anterior circulation aneurysms. The approach does expose a wide variety of critical structures, placing them at risk for inadvertent injury. Nevertheless, we have used this approach in multiple cases and have enjoyed the ability to visualize the basilar apex from the front (allowing for easier exploration of the contralateral PCA and its perforators) as well as from a more lateral view (allowing for excellent dissection of the perforators running behind a larger apex aneurysm).

No matter which approach is chosen, once the clip has been applied, the surgeon must painstakingly inspect the basilar apex to be certain no perforators have been compromised (**Table 7.1**).

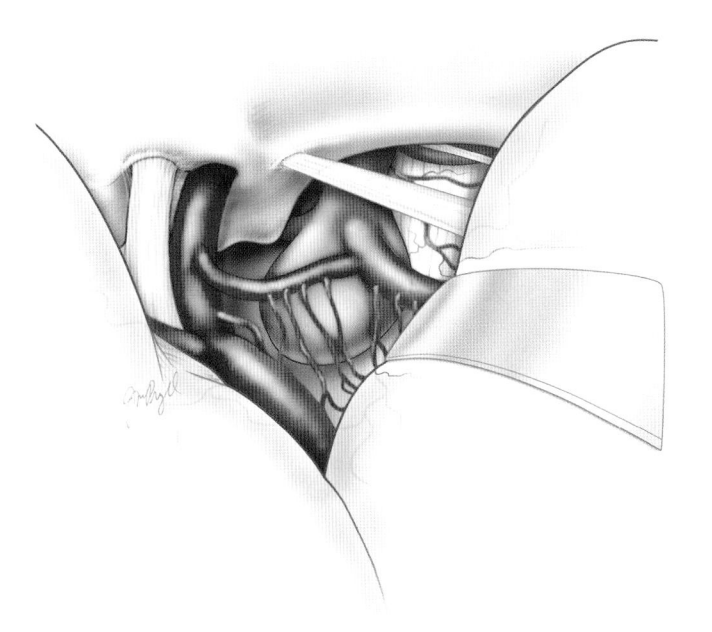

Fig. 7.9 Artist's illustration of a "half-half" approach demonstrating the compromise exposure between the pterional and subtemporal approaches. Note the visibility of the opposite P1, along with the option of working from a more lateral perspective behind the aneurysm.

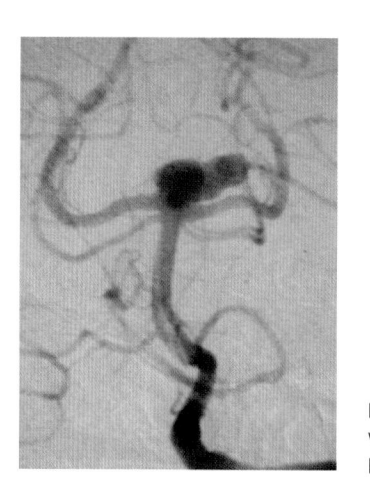

Fig. 7.10   A large, irregular basilar apex aneurysm, which was explored and clipped through a half-half approach as shown in ⟳ VIDEO 39 .

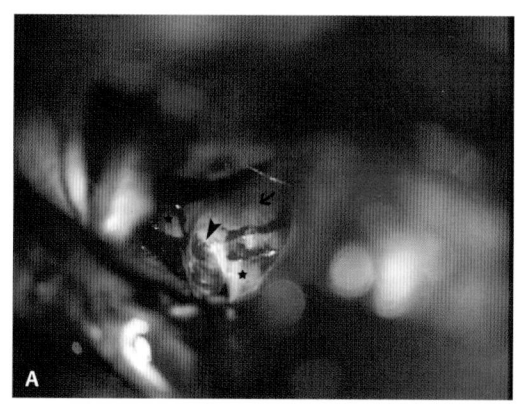

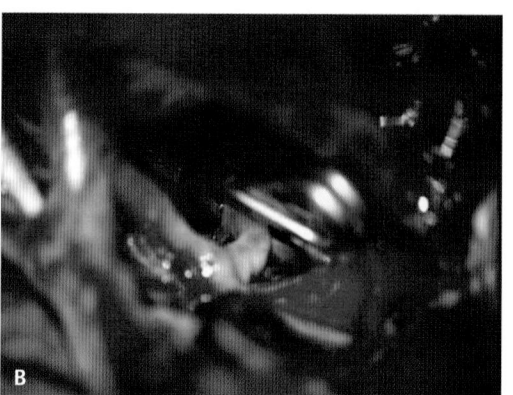

Fig. 7.11   (A) A small, thin-walled basilar apex aneurysm (*arrowhead*) is exposed along with the upper basilar artery (*arrow*) and both P1 segments (*stars*). **(B)** The aneurysm has been repaired with a fenestrated clip around the P1.

Table 7.1 ■ **Basilar Apex Aneurysm Pearls and Pitfalls**

This is the most difficult of the standard aneurysm locations.

Consider endovascular therapy if feasible.

Consider referral to high-volume center if surgery required.

Pterional, half-half, subtemporal approaches may be used.

Orbitozygomatic osteotomy may be helpful.

Consider anterior clinoid removal with mobilization of optic nerve.

Evaluate relationship to posterior clinoid on preoperative angiography—a very high or very low basilar apex represents a surgical challenge.

Use a ventriculostomy or lumbar drain in the setting of subarachnoid hemorrhage.

Lumbar drain is helpful for subtemporal approach in unruptured setting.

Follow ipsilateral P1 back to bifurcation to reach aneurysm.

The surgeon must have good visualization despite narrow working corridor.

The surgeon must preserve all perforating vessels.

Posteriorly directed lesions can be buried in brainstem and are most dangerous and difficult.

Intraoperative angiography is needed to avoid inadvertent vascular compromise.

Ipsilateral PCommA can be sacrificed to widen tight exposure, but this will limit collateral supply, so we avoid sacrificing a large PCommA in this setting.

Never sacrifice a fetal PCommA.

Be gentle on third nerve to avoid significant palsy.

Divide and suture back tent just behind entry of fourth nerve into tentorial edge to widen working angle, particularly for subtemporal approach.

Temporary clips are very helpful for basilar apex aneurysms.

Fenestrated clips are often useful, placing ipsilateral P1 in fenestration.

Be flexible in the operating room if unexpected intraoperative findings suggest the situation may be more complicated than initially anticipated.

Perforator injury can result in severe neurological deficit.

■ Superior Cerebellar Artery Aneurysms

Aneurysms arising between the PCA and SCA origins along the upper basilar artery are significantly easier to treat surgically than true apex lesions. Pterional or subtemporal exposures can be used as just discussed. As with basilar apex lesions, the surgeon should preserve all perforators arising from the basilar artery, the proximal PCA, or the SCA. In our experience, the SCA origin is often incorporated into the aneurysm base but can usually be reconstructed by strategic clip placement. In our practice, we have generally used a simple pterional approach for most of these lesions, although larger aneurysms may require a more extensive exposure ⏵ VIDEO 40) (**Figs. 7.12, 7.13**). The third nerve, which also runs between the PCA and SCA, can be injured during exposure and clipping of these lesions ⏵ VIDEO 41) (**Table 7.2**).

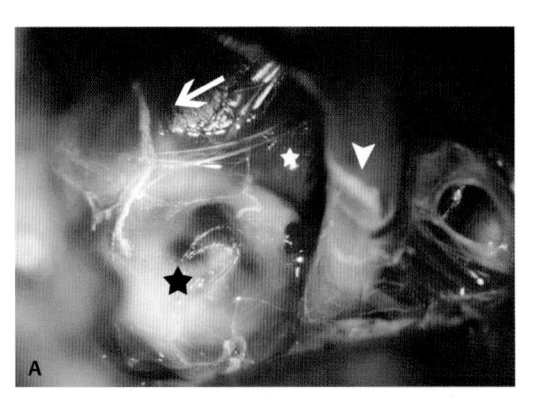

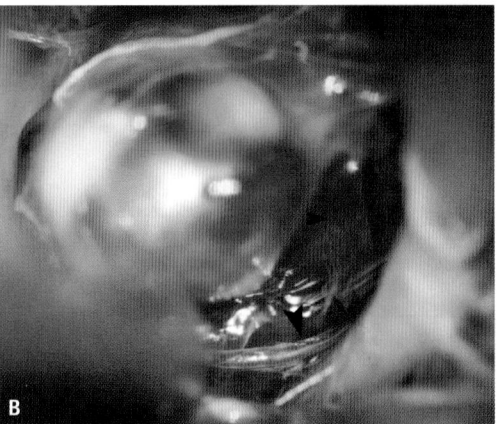

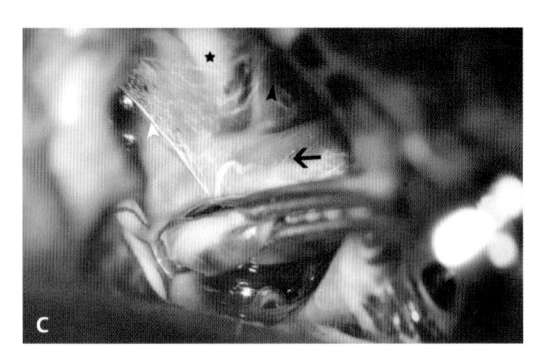

Fig. 7.12 **(A)** A broad-based aneurysm (*star*) of the upper BA (*white arrow*) is exposed just above the third cranial nerve (*white arrowhead*). Note the origin of the SCA (*white star*), which arises from the inferior neck of the aneurysm. **(B)** Perforators (*arrowheads*) are dissected from the back wall of the aneurysm prior to clipping. **(C)** A curved clip has been used to reconstruct the sidewall of the upper BA (*arrow*). The opposite SCA (*black arrowhead*), third cranial nerve (*black star*), and PCA (*white arrowhead*) are visible.

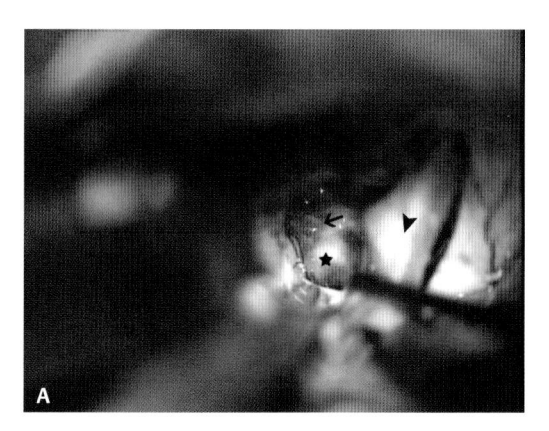

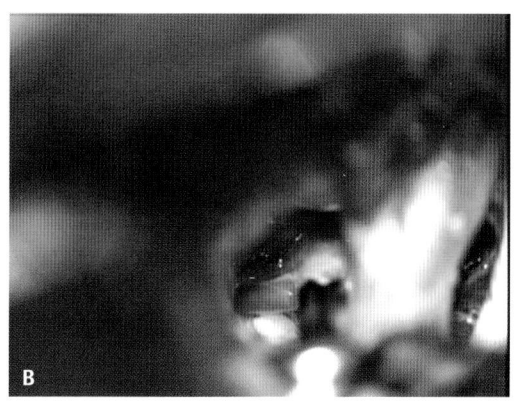

Fig. 7.13 **(A)** A small aneurysm (*star*) arising at the origin of the SCA (*arrow*) is exposed by retracting the ICA (*arrowhead*) medially. **(B)** The aneurysm has been clipped.

Table 7.2 ■ **SCA Aneurysm Pearls and Pitfalls**

Approaches are the same as for basilar apex aneurysms.

Protect perforators off basilar artery, P1, SCA.

Watch the origin of the SCA, which may be incorporated into neck of the aneurysm.

The aneurysm dome may be adherent to the third nerve in larger aneurysms.

◼ Basilar Trunk and Vertebrobasilar Junction Aneurysms

Aneurysms involving the basilar trunk are rare. They may represent dissections or may be truly saccular in nature. One video of such a lesion treated via a presigmoid-subtemporal approach has been included in this work for viewer interest ⏵ VIDEO 42 (**Fig. 7.14**). We have found this approach to give the widest working angle for such lesions and have treated a half-dozen similar lesions using this surgical trajectory. The choice of approach in these cases will depend on the regional

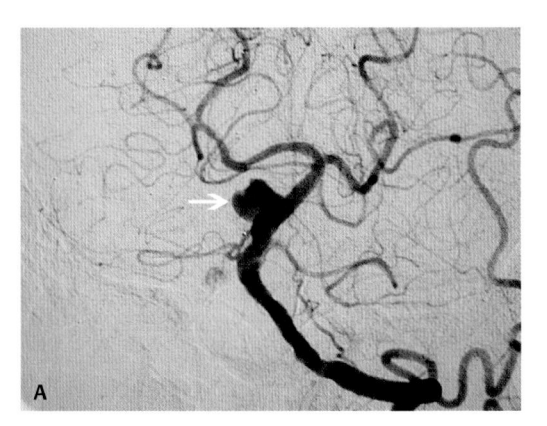

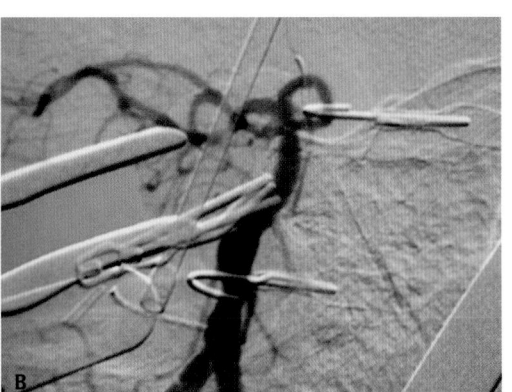

Fig. 7.14   (A) A preoperative arteriogram demonstrates an unusual sidewall aneurysm (arrow) of the basilar trunk. This lesion was exposed and treated using a combined presigmoid-subtemporal approach. **(B)** Intraoperative angiogram demonstrates occlusion of the aneurysm. The treatment of this lesion is seen in ⏵ VIDEO 42 .

anatomy. In some instances, particularly when the aneurysm is sitting at or above the level of the tentorium, an OZ or subtemporal approach may be sufficient. More commonly, the lesion is situated lower in the posterior fossa, and an approach that offers wide access to the cerebellopontine angle and affords proximal control of the lower basilar artery is useful.

Also included in this category are lesions of the vertebrobasilar junction. We have treated the majority of these lesions endovascularly because of the difficulty associated with surgically accessing this location. Vertebrobasilar junction aneurysms are often multilobulated, may be associated with a fenestration of the proximal basilar artery, and frequently present with rupture. We have used a far lateral suboccipital approach when treating these lesions surgically (**Fig. 7.15**). The details of this approach will be described more fully in Chapter 8, which details the treatment of posterior inferior cerebellar artery (PICA) aneurysms (**Table 7.3**).

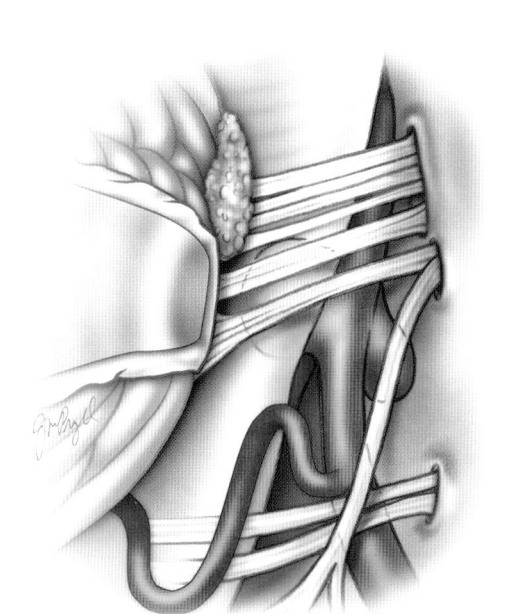

Fig. 7.15 Artist's illustration of a far lateral suboccipital approach with gentle cerebellar retraction to expose a multilobulated vertebrobasilar junction aneurysm. The surgeon must work past the fine lower cranial nerve rootlets to reach the aneurysm, which may be directed ventrally toward the clivus or back toward the brainstem.

Table 7.3 ■ **Basilar Trunk Aneurysm Pearls and Pitfalls**

These aneurysms are rare.

They may represent dissections, and thus may be dynamic and unstable.

Proximal control of lower basilar artery is important.

The surgeon must be able to visualize and dissect aneurysm away from brainstem.

Liberal use of skull base approaches, as needed, has been helpful to us.

Carefully visualize all brainstem perforators.

The surgeon must work past multiple cranial nerves, which should be carefully protected.

Brainstem and/or cerebellar ischemia may result from inadvertent occlusion of perforators or major branch vessels.

CSF fistula may occur from open mastoid air cells.

Use far lateral suboccipital approach for lower basilar trunk and vertebrobasilar junction aneurysms.

Endovascular therapy is useful for most vertebrobasilar junction aneurysms.

8 Posterior Inferior Cerebellar Artery Aneurysms

Posterior inferior cerebellar artery (PICA) aneurysms are relatively uncommon. Most PICA aneurysms can be treated endovascularly, but we have encountered a high rate of aneurysm recurrence associated with coiling procedures. As a result, surgical consideration should be given to PICA aneurysms, particularly those with wider necks. The classic PICA aneurysm arises at the takeoff of the PICA from the vertebral artery. These aneurysms can be challenging because of the great variability of the local vascular anatomy. At times, the aneurysm can be located along the antero-lateral surface of the medulla and even as high as the cerebellopontine angle. We have found it useful to study the preoperative angiogram to determine the location of the aneurysm relative to the skull base when deciding how difficult the surgical exposure will be (**Fig. 8.1**).

Many PICA aneurysms occur close to the point where the vertebral artery penetrates the dura not far above the craniocervical junction. These cases can be exposed in straightforward fashion, and distal control of the vertebral artery can be achieved without difficulty (**Fig. 8.2**). In our experience, when the PICA takes origin from the vertebral artery low on its vertical segment, the aneurysm will generally be closer to the foramen magnum. On the other hand, when the PICA arises at the turn of the artery where it becomes horizontal or along its horizontal segment just before the vertebrobasilar junction, the surgeon can anticipate a more challenging exposure (**Fig. 8.3**).

We use a far lateral suboccipital approach for these lesions (**Figs. 8.4, 8.5**). The patient can be prone, lateral, or three-quarters prone, depending on the surgeon's preference. As part of the exposure, we drill down the condyle aggressively to op-

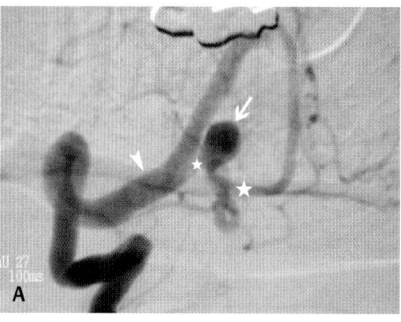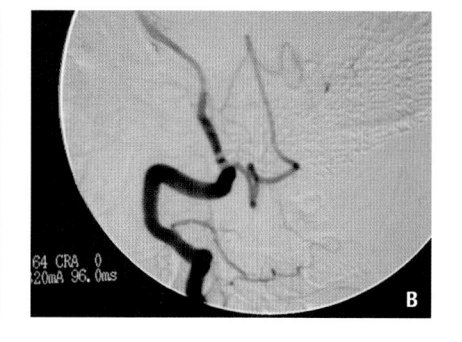

Fig. 8.1 **(A)** Vertebral arteriogram demonstrates a somewhat fusiform aneurysm (*arrow*) arising just distal to the PICA origin (*small white star*) on the PICA itself (*larger white star*). The PICA origin is low on the vertical portion of the vertebral artery (*arrowhead*), presumably close to the location where the artery becomes intradural. This suggests an easier exposure. **(B)** Postoperative arteriogram demonstrates clip occlusion of the aneurysm.

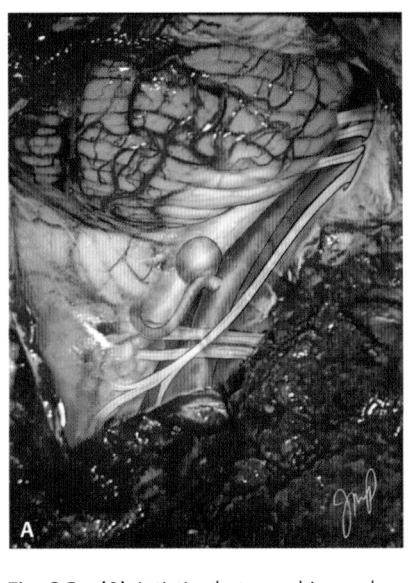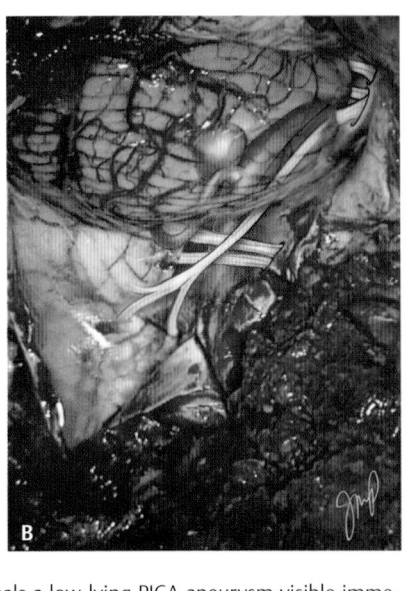

Fig. 8.2 **(A)** Artist's photographic overlay reveals a low-lying PICA aneurysm visible immediately after dural opening without cerebellar retraction. **(B)** A more common situation is shown, in which a PICA aneurysm is initially hidden by the cerebellum.

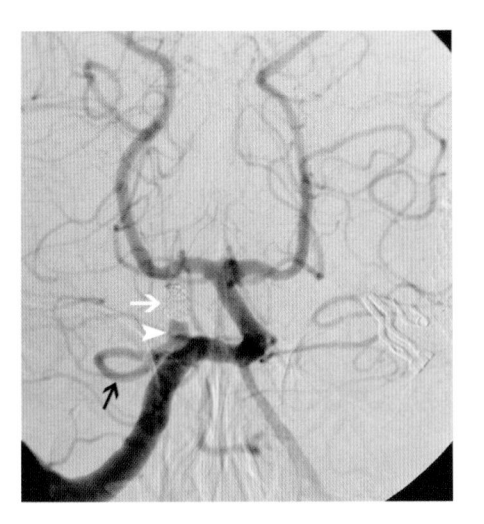

Fig. 8.3 Vertebral arteriogram demonstrates recurrent PICA aneurysm (*white arrowhead*) with a coil mass (*white arrow*) displaced upward within the aneurysm. The PICA (*black arrow*) arises at the aneurysm neck. Note the location of the aneurysm high on the vertebral artery, where the artery has become horizontal and is curving to reach the vertebrobasilar junction. This was treated through a far lateral suboccipital approach and was technically more difficult than the case shown in **Fig. 8.1**.

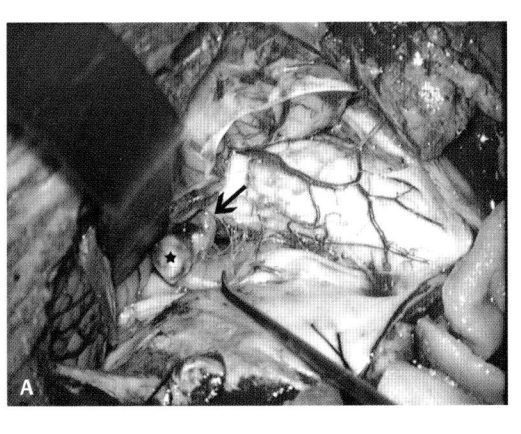

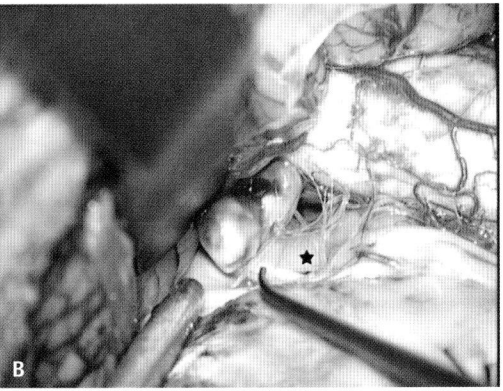

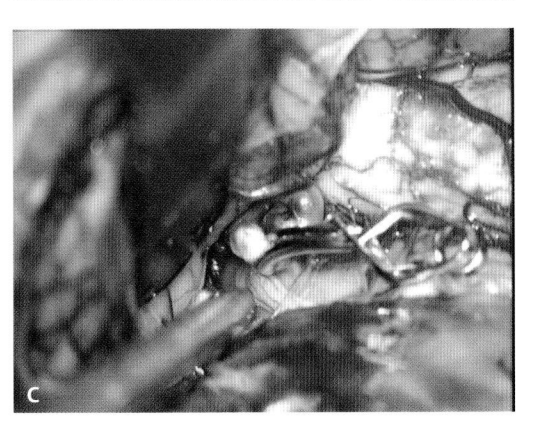

Fig. 8.4 **(A)** A far lateral suboccipital approach has been completed. The dura is reflected back and an excellent exposure of the lower medulla with its associated anatomy is provided. By gently elevating the cerebellum, the vertebral artery (proximal and distal to the PICA) is seen along with the aneurysm (*star*), the PICA itself (*arrow*), and lower cranial nerve rootlets. **(B)** In this magnified view, the proximal intradural vertebral artery (*star*) is appreciated. **(C)** The aneurysm has been repaired with a single clip.

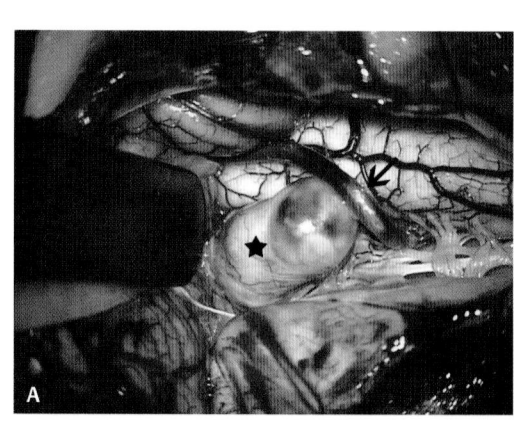

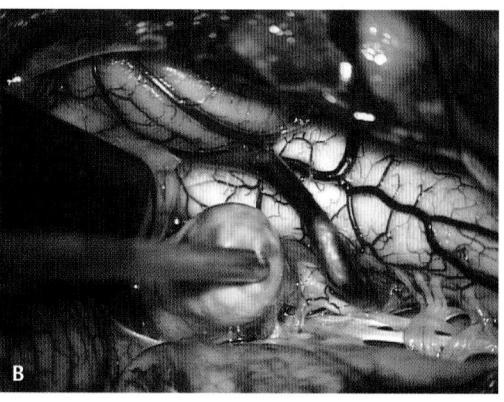

Fig. 8.5 **(A)** A large, atheromatous PICA aneurysm (*star*) is exposed **(A)** with a more normal-appearing PICA (*arrow*) emerging from its base. **(B)** The aneurysm is reflected upward to reveal the underlying vertebral artery and PICA origin.

timize visualization of the critical intradural anatomy. The vertebral artery is readily exposed extradurally along the lateral aspect of the C1 arch, where hemostatic agents may be useful in controlling bothersome venous bleeding from the vertebral venous plexus. Once the dura is opened, the intradural vertebral artery can be traced to the PICA origin, offering early proximal control (**Fig. 8.6**). Gentle retraction of the cerebellar tonsil may be helpful with exposure. When the distal vertebral artery communicates normally with the vertebrobasilar junction, retrograde bleeding from the opposite vertebral artery can be problematic should the aneurysm rupture intraoperatively. Therefore, in the setting of a recent rupture, we expose the vertebral artery distal to the PICA origin to obtain proximal and distal control prior to dissection of the aneurysm .

While exposing a PICA aneurysm, the surgeon will typically work past the fine and delicate lower cranial nerve rootlets (**Fig. 8.7**). In the unruptured setting, these

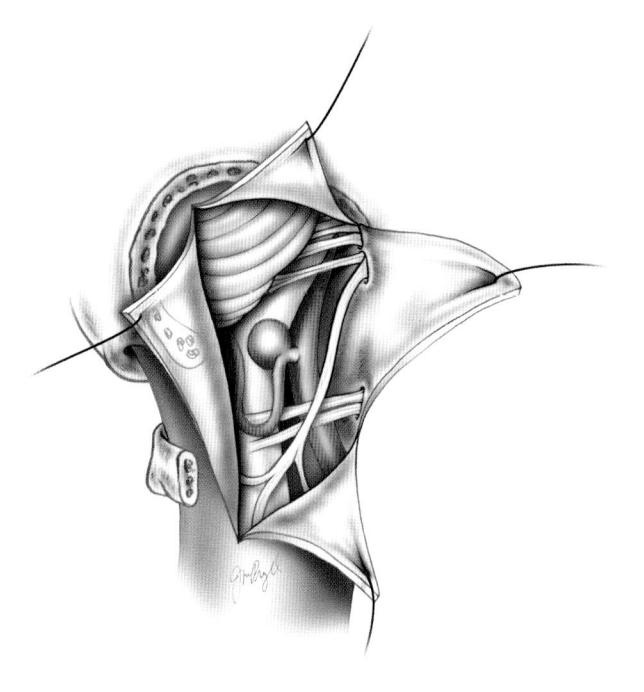

Fig. 8.6 Artist's illustration depicting a far lateral suboccipital approach. The dura has been opened to reveal a PICA-origin aneurysm along the lateral aspect of the medulla. Lower cranial nerves are seen crossing the field.

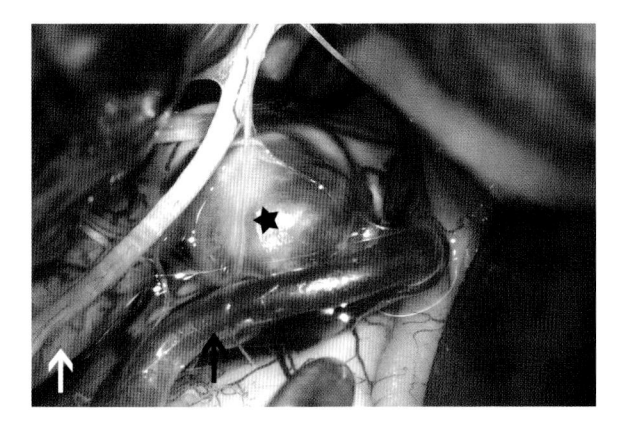

Fig. 8.7 A PICA aneurysm (*star*) and the associated PICA (*black arrow*) have been exposed with cranial nerve XI as well as fine rootlets of the other lower cranial nerves crossing the field. The vertebral artery (*white arrow*) has been exposed proximal to the PICA origin.

can be easily identified and preserved, but in the setting of a subarachnoid hemorrhage (SAH), it can be more difficult to protect these rootlets when they are encased in thick subarachnoid clot. In all instances, the nerves should be carefully protected during surgery, and we generally test patients for ipsilateral swallowing difficulty prior to initiating a regular diet postoperatively.

We have included several examples of PICA aneurysms in this series to illustrate their surgical treatment ⏩ VIDEO 43 ⏩ VIDEO 44 ⏩ VIDEO 45 (**Figs. 8.8, 8.9**).

It should be noted that if formal digital subtraction angiography is planned as an intraoperative measure during the treatment of a PICA aneurysm, the preoperative placement of a long femoral sheath is strongly recommended, as the patient is typically positioned such that it would be awkward or impossible to place the sheath once the procedure is under way (**Table 8.1**).

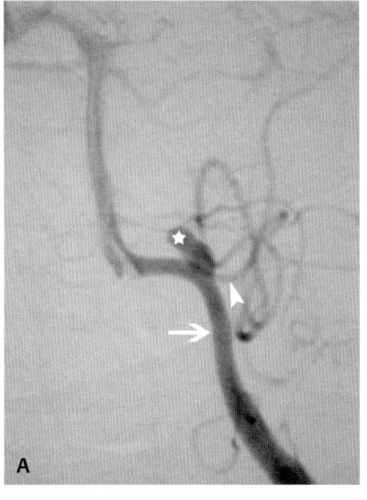 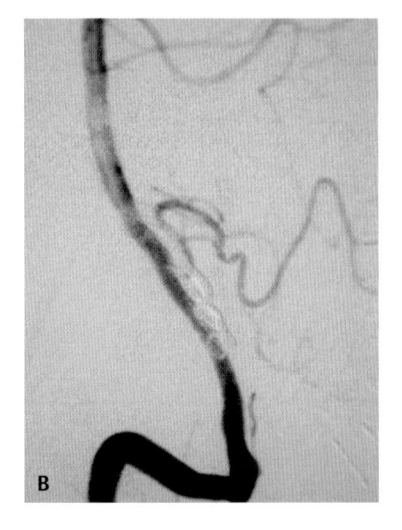

Fig. 8.8 **(A)** Vertebral angiography demonstrates a PICA aneurysm (*star*) arising high on the vertebral artery (*arrow*) at the start of its horizontal intracranial segment. The PICA (*arrowhead*) is readily appreciated. **(B)** The aneurysm has been occluded with a fenestrated clip. The treatment of this lesion is shown in ⏩ VIDEO 44 .

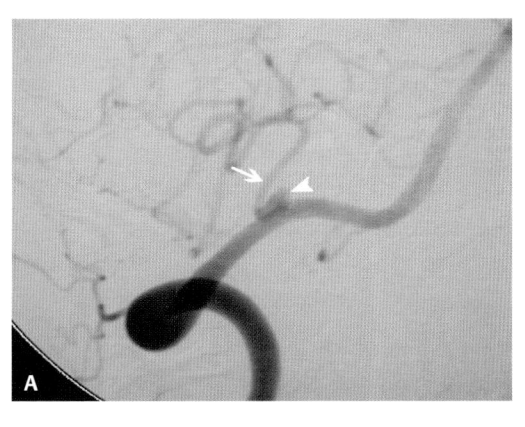

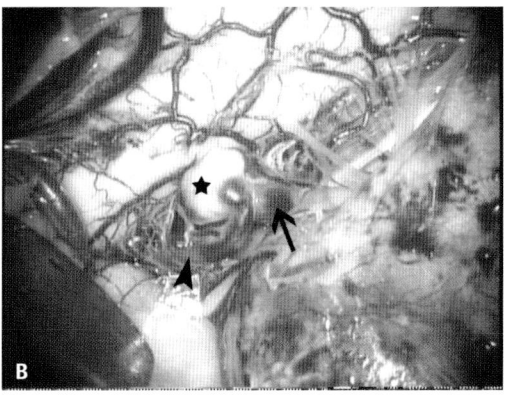

Fig. 8.9 **(A)** Preoperative vertebral arteriogram shows a small PICA aneurysm (*arrowhead*) in a young patient with multiple aneurysms. The PICA (*arrow*) arises from the base of the aneurysm. **(B)** The lesion is exposed through a far lateral suboccipital approach, and the proximal vertebral artery (*arrow*), aneurysm (*star*), and PICA (*arrowhead*) are readily seen. The treatment of this lesion is shown in ◀ VIDEO 45 .

Table 8.1   ■   PICA Aneurysm Pearls and Pitfalls

Use the far lateral suboccipital approach.

Remove adequate amount of the occipital condyle for visualization.

Identify intradural vertebral artery for proximal control.

Trace vertebral artery to PICA origin.

Expose distal vertebral as well for complete control of aneurysm.

Watch for exposed mastoid air cells to avoid delayed CSF fistula or infection.

Gently elevate cerebellar tonsil as needed.

Carefully protect fine lower cranial nerve rootlets; injury to rootlets may cause dysphagia or dysphonia.

Be particularly cautious with rootlets encased in thick subarachnoid clot.

Be aware of high-lying aneurysms, which can be difficult to reach.

PICA infarct can result in Wallenberg syndrome: ataxia, dysphagia, dysarthria, vertigo, nystagmus, Horner syndrome, sensory disturbance.

Place long femoral sheath preoperatively if an intraoperative digital subtraction angiogram is planned.

9 Special Considerations: Giant Aneurysms, Bypasses, Previously Coiled Lesions, and Rare Locations

Giant Aneurysms

Giant aneurysms, defined as lesions measuring at least 2.5 cm in maximal dimension, demand great technical expertise and creativity if a surgeon hopes to achieve good results in a reliable fashion. There is no one method to treat these complex lesions, and the exact technique chosen must depend heavily on the specific situation. If local mass effect is a significant issue, then some treatment that will enable emptying and deflation of the lesion should be considered. This may include direct clipping, aneurysmorrhaphy with reconstruction, or trapping with distal revascularization. When mass effect is not a problem, a simple parent artery occlusion with distal revascularization may be sufficient. Although cranial neuropathy resulting from local pressure exerted by a small aneurysm has been shown to resolve with endovascular therapy, we have considered such compression in the setting of a giant aneurysm an indication for open surgical decompression.

In truth, an entire book could be written focusing on the management of giant aneurysms. In most cases, simple neck clipping will not be feasible. When attempting direct clipping, the thick necks of these aneurysms will often preclude simple clips from closing. The surgeon must be very careful to avoid creating a tear at the junction of the neck with the parent artery or an efferent branch as a large heavy clip attempts to force shut a thickened neck that resists closure. Although surgical exploration for possible clipping is often worthwhile, the surgeon should have a well-measured plan of attack that assumes attempted primary clip reconstruction may be unsuccessful.

When evaluating giant aneurysms, several points should always be considered. These include: patient age and comorbidities, the presence or absence of symptomatic mass effect, degree of calcification and atheroma at the aneurysm neck based on cross-sectional imaging, incorporation of efferent branches into the aneurysm neck, likely tolerance of temporary or permanent occlusion, possible role of bypass, size of the superficial temporal artery (STA) and occipital artery, and potential tolerance of deep hypothermic arrest.

Despite the inherent challenges, some giant aneurysms can be clipped primarily, and surgical exploration to attempt primary clipping represents a reasonable approach in selected cases (**Figs. 9.1, 9.2**). Adjunctive techniques that we have found useful or essential in these cases include the liberal use of temporary clips, suction decompression, deep hypothermic circulatory arrest, and preliminary bypass to allow for prolonged temporary occlusion.

The first video in this chapter demonstrates the treatment of a giant ruptured paraclinoid aneurysm repaired using multiple fenestrated clips to reconstruct the internal carotid artery (ICA) during a short period of temporary occlusion (VIDEO 46). If the aneurysm in this case had not softened considerably with simple temporary clipping, then suction decompression could have been utilized.

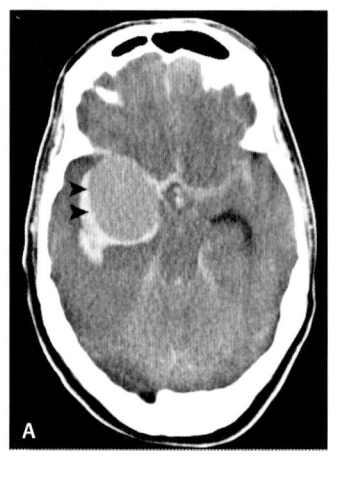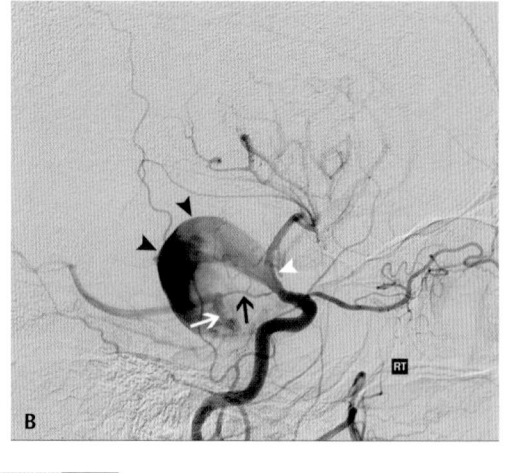

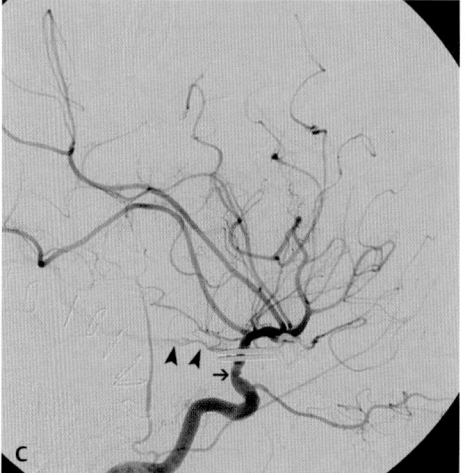

Fig. 9.1 **(A)** Axial CT scan demonstrates a diffuse subarachnoid hemorrhage (SAH) resulting from a truly giant aneurysm (*arrowheads*) with surrounding hematoma displacing the right temporal lobe. **(B)** A giant aneurysm (*black arrowheads*) arising from the posterior wall of the supraclinoid internal carotid artery (ICA) (*white arrowhead*) is identified on this lateral internal carotid arteriogram. Note the posterior communicating artery (*black arrow*) seen filling behind the aneurysm to irrigate the upper basilar artery (BA) (*white arrow*) and posterior cerebral artery (PCA). The patient was brought to the operating room on an urgent basis, and the aneurysm was repaired using a ten-minute period of temporary trapping of the supraclinoid ICA. **(C)** A postoperative lateral carotid arteriogram demonstrates occlusion of the aneurysm with a single long clip. Note the preservation of the posterior communicating artery (PCommA) (*arrowheads*). Moderate vasospasm of the supraclinoid ICA is noted (*arrow*).

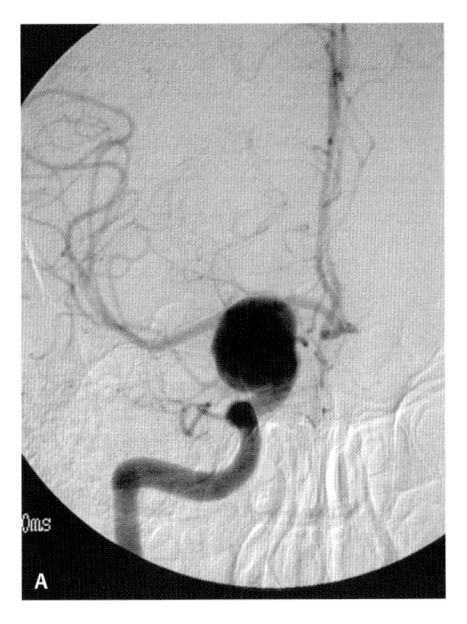

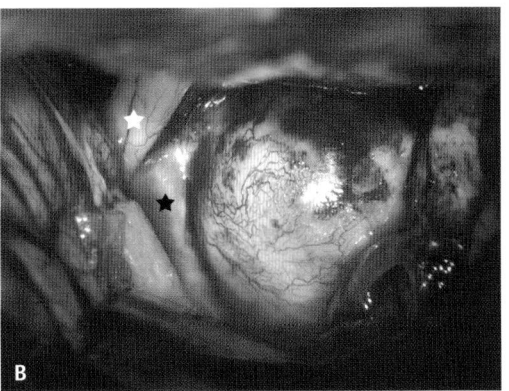

Fig. 9.2 **(A)** Anteroposterior right internal carotid arteriogram demonstrates a partially thrombosed giant aneurysm arising from the supraclinoid internal carotid artery. **(B)** Intraoperative photomicrograph reveals the giant aneurysm with forward displacement of the internal carotid artery (*black star*) and optic nerve (*white star*). *(Continued on page 102)*

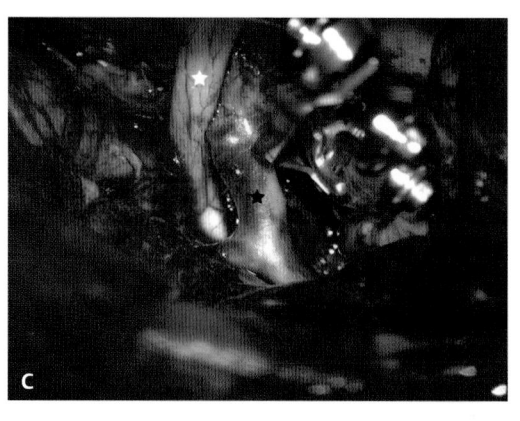

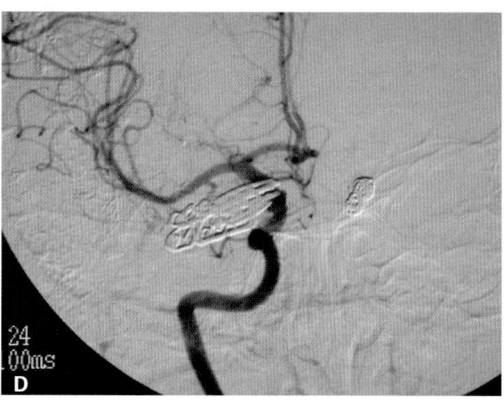

Fig. 9.2 *(Continued)* **(C)** The lesion has been reconstructed with multiple clips, and the internal carotid artery (*black star*) and optic nerve (*white star*) have regained a more normal appearance with the mass effect relieved. **(D)** Postoperative anteroposterior internal carotid arteriogram demonstrates occlusion of the aneurysm

In some cases, it appears that the aneurysm will be clippable, but only with a period of prolonged temporary occlusion that will likely exceed the patient's tolerance for such occlusion. In these instances, we have utilized either deep hypothermic circulatory arrest or preliminary bypass to enable the prolonged occlusion.

In the most experienced of hands, deep hypothermic circulatory arrest procedures carry significant morbidity and mortality, exceeding 10% for the systemic complications relating to the cardiac procedure alone. Nevertheless, in selected instances, circulatory arrest will allow the surgeon the time necessary to properly dissect and clip a giant aneurysm. The cardiac surgeon can provide a "low-flow state" during which the preliminary dissection can be completed, leaving only the final critical stages of the dissection and clipping for the true arrest period. The arrest can be performed using either a closed- or open-chest technique, and periods of arrest exceeding one hour have been utilized safely and successfully. Nevertheless, we have preferred to keep the arrest period under 45 minutes whenever possible.

When performing an arrest procedure, the craniotomy opening should be meticulous in terms of hemostasis, as the patient will be fully anticoagulated for a prolonged period and the hypothermia will further compromise clotting. It is quite amazing to watch complete cessation of blood flow to the brain. As pulsation stops, the intracranial circulation empties, allowing for aggressive dissection of the aneurysm. Once the aneurysm has been clipped, the neurosurgeon must wait during the rewarming process prior to closing the craniotomy. Only when the heparin has been fully reversed and normal coagulation has been restored can the craniotomy be closed. We have included one example of a deep hypothermic circulatory arrest for a giant ruptured anterior communicating artery (ACommA) aneurysm with severe subarachnoid hemorrhage (SAH) 🔵 VIDEO 47) (**Fig. 9.3**).

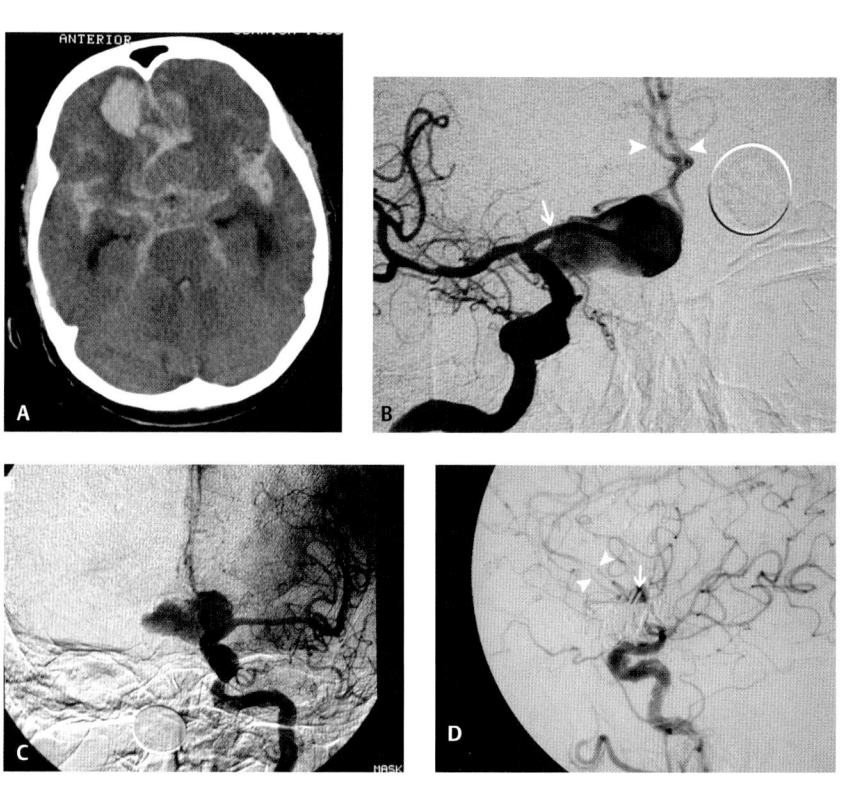

Fig. 9.3   **(A)** A severe subarachnoid hemorrhage is seen on the axial CT scan. **(B)** Right internal carotid arteriogram reveals a giant multilobulated ACommA aneurysm. The A1 (*arrow*) and A2 vessels (*arrowheads*) are seen. **(C)** Left carotid arteriogram demonstrates an additional component to the aneurysm. Only by studying the right and left arteriographic injections simultaneously does one obtain a full appreciation of the extent of the aneurysm. This lesion was treated using deep hypothermic circulatory arrest as shown in 🔵 VIDEO 47). **(D)** Immediate postoperative angiographic image shows residual fullness (*arrow*) in the region of the anterior communicating artery which was left to preserve filling of the A2 vessels (*arrowheads*).

To illustrate the use of preliminary bypass to enable prolonged temporary occlusion, we have included an example of a giant carotid ophthalmic aneurysm managed in this fashion, using a superficial temporal artery to middle cerebral artery (STA-MCA) bypass ⏵VIDEO 48 (**Fig. 9.4**). The advantage of this technique includes the possibility of using permanent occlusion as a treatment option if the aneurysm cannot be primarily reconstructed. Nevertheless, the bypass takes time at the beginning of an already challenging procedure, and this must be weighed when considering the various treatment options.

When a giant aneurysm cannot be clipped primarily, we have found the use of various bypass techniques to be incredibly helpful in managing even the most complex of giant aneurysms. Multiple examples of such cases are included in the next section.

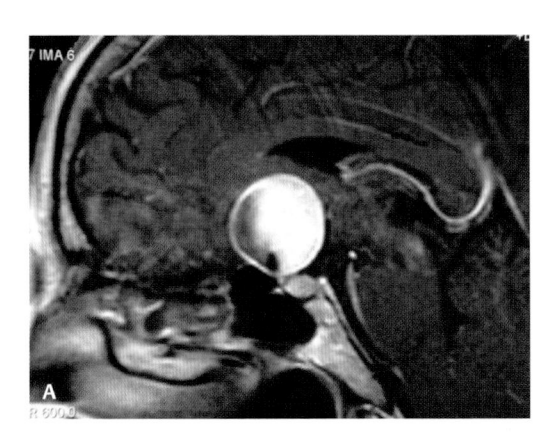

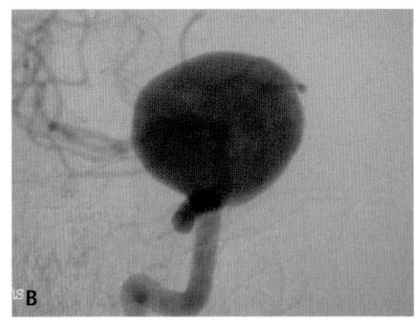
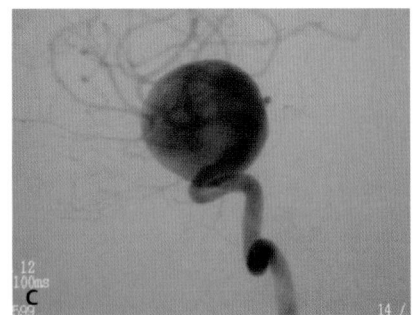

Fig. 9.4 **(A)** A sagittal MR image reveals a giant aneurysm in the suprasellar region. **(B)** Anteroposterior internal carotid arteriogram shows a truly giant paraclinoid aneurysm. **(C)** Corresponding lateral angiographic image. This lesion was treated with preliminary double-barrel bypass to allow prolonged temporary occlusion, which then enabled proper clipping of the aneurysm.

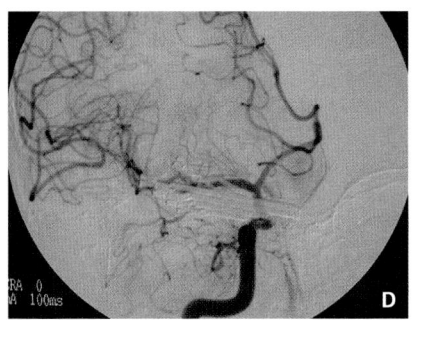 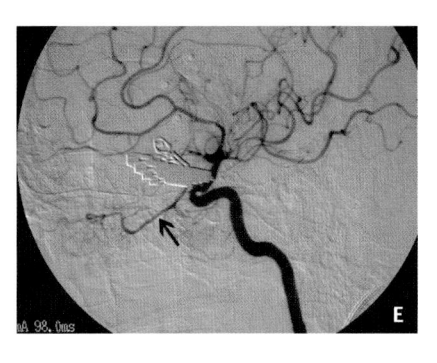

Fig. 9.4 *(Continued)*   **(D)** Postoperative arteriogram reveals complete occlusion of the aneurysm with preservation of the normal vasculature. **(E)** Lateral arteriogram shows the reconstruction and highlights preservation of the ophthalmic artery *(arrow)*. The treatment of this lesion can be seen in VIDEO 48 .

Bypass for "Unclippable" Aneurysms

The judicious use of bypass procedures to treat intracranial aneurysms can allow even a young surgeon to treat the most daunting of aneurysms. Although there are some surgeons who can successfully clip a giant basilar aneurysm, we have used bypass and occlusion in such cases to achieve a good result without having to dissect the fine perforators from behind these difficult lesions. Similarly, a distal bypass and parent artery occlusion represent an excellent option for dealing with many giant aneurysms that have atheromatous or calcified walls and are filled with organized clot or coils.

The exact form of bypass will depend on the specifics of the case. When replacing the ICA, a preoperative balloon occlusion test is useful to assess the degree of collateral flow and determine whether a low-flow STA-MCA bypass or a higher-flow radial artery or saphenous vein graft is appropriate. When collateral is robust, and particularly in an older patient, a simple occlusion without revascularization can be considered. When occluding a more distal artery, we have used a variety of creative revascularization options followed by trapping or parent artery occlusion for an "unclippable" aneurysm. Excision with end-to-end reanastomosis, vascular reimplantation, short intracranial-intracranial jump grafts, side-to-side anastomosis, and more traditional extracranial-intracranial (EC-IC) bypass have all been used with success in such cases.

Multiple examples of the use of various bypass techniques and strategies are included in VIDEO 49   VIDEO 50   VIDEO 51 (**Figs. 9.5–9.9**).

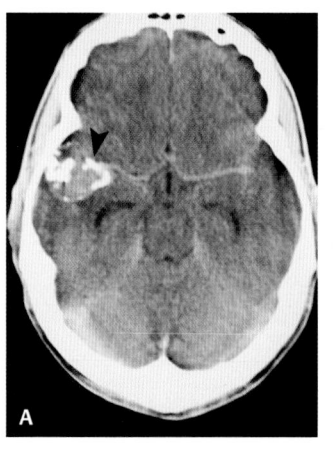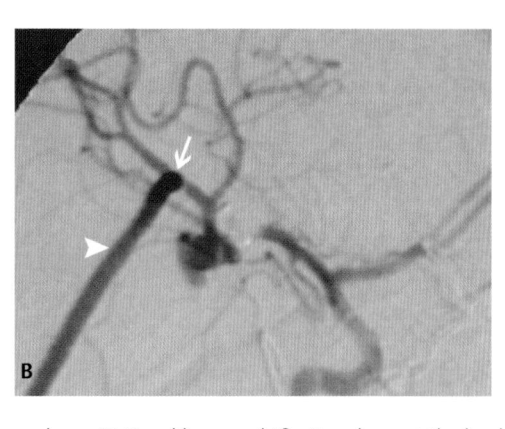

Fig. 9.5 **(A)** Preoperative axial CT scan shows SAH and heavy calcification down at the level of the neck of a giant MCA aneurysm (*arrowhead*) in a young patient. The lesion was treated using a radial artery graft. **(B)** An intraoperative angiogram demonstrates filling of the entire MCA territory as well as the aneurysm through the radial artery graft (*arrowhead*). The site of the distal anastomosis is shown (*arrow*). The treatment of this lesion is included in ⏵ VIDEO 49 .

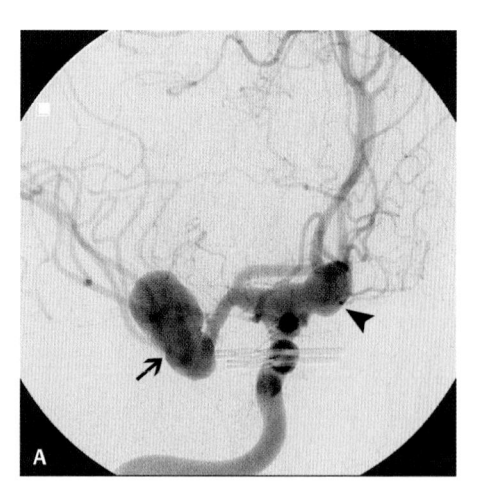

Fig. 9.6 **(A)** A giant MCA aneurysm (*arrow*) with an associated fusiform supraclinoid ICA aneurysm (*arrowhead*) is shown on an anteroposterior angiogram.

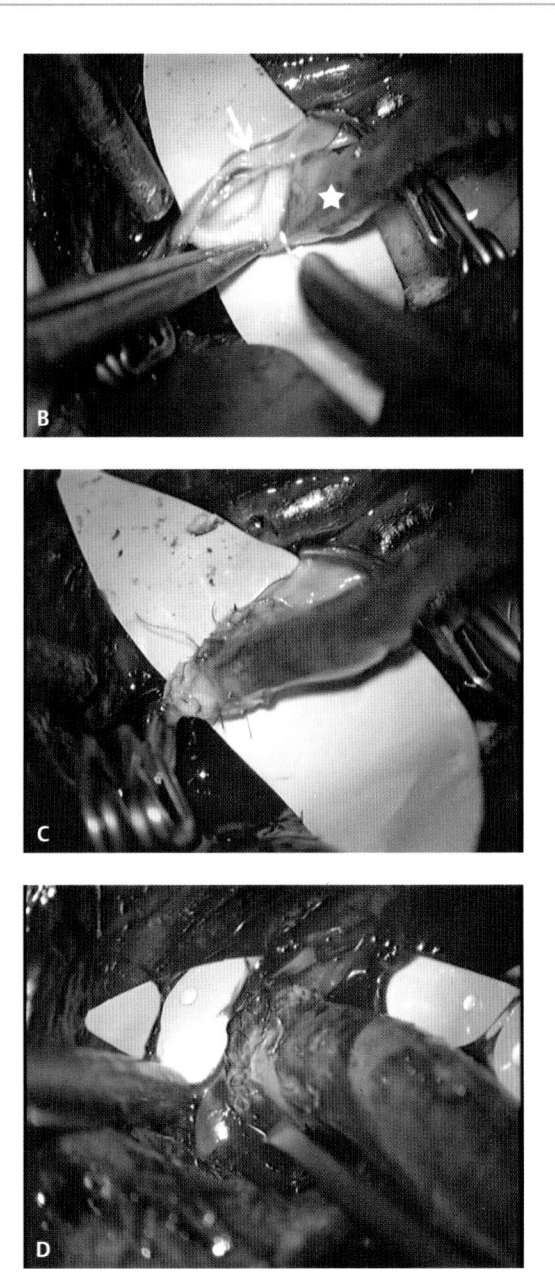

Fig. 9.6 *(Continued)*   **(B)** Intraoperative photomicrograph showing the distal anastomosis of a long saphenous vein graft *(star)* being sewn to a middle cerebral branch *(arrow)*. **(C)** The anastomosis has been completed. **(D)** The clips have been removed. *(Continued on page 108)*

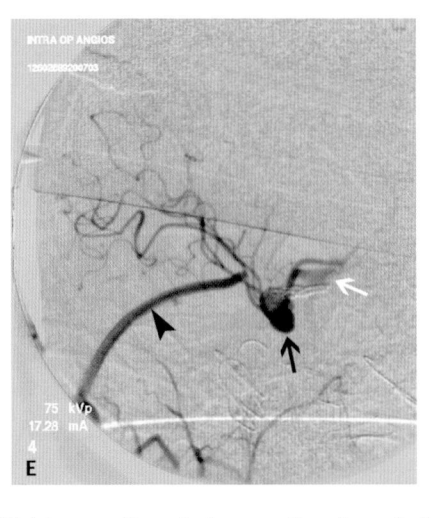

Fig. 9.6 *(Continued)* **(E)** Intraoperative arteriogram after clip occlusion of the distal supra-clinoid internal carotid artery demonstrates immediate decreased filling of both the middle cerebral aneurysm (*black arrow*) and the fusiform internal carotid aneurysm (*white arrow*) with excellent filling of the long vein graft (*arrowhead*).

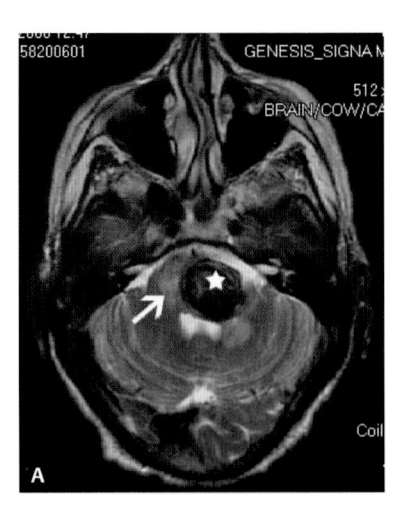

Fig. 9.7 **(A)** A giant PICA aneurysm (*star*) is shown on an axial MR image with significant brainstem compression and local edema (*white arrow*).

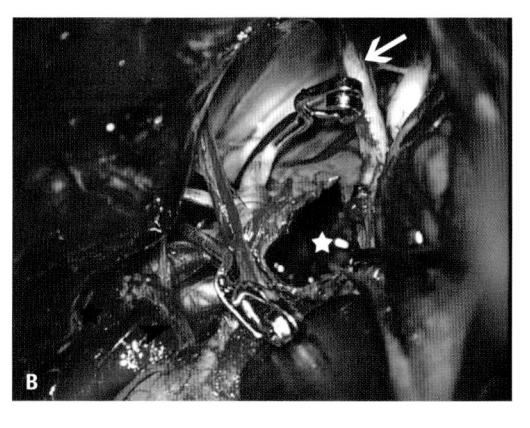

Fig. 9.7 *(Continued)* **(B)** The lesion has been exposed through a far lateral suboccipital approach. The PICA (*arrowhead*) has been cut at its origin from the thick-walled aneurysm and reimplanted onto the more proximal vertebral artery (*black star*), allowing us to trap and evacuate the aneurysm (*white star*) of thrombus. Note the clips on the vertebral artery proximal and distal to the aneurysm, the view into the opened and evacuated aneurysm (*white star*), and the seventh-eighth cranial nerve complex (*white arrow*).

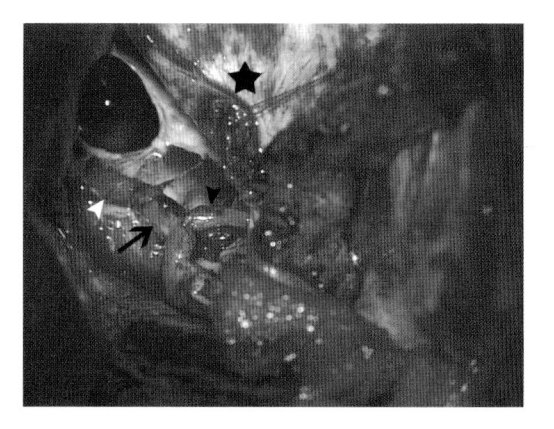

Fig. 9.8 Using a subtemporal approach, a generous superficial temporal artery has been anastomosed to the PCA on the side of the brainstem to enable treatment of a giant fusiform basilar artery (BA) aneurysm. Note the long, flat anastomosis (*black arrow*), the PCA proximal (*white arrowhead*) and distal (*black arrowhead*) to the anastomosis, and the tentorium (*black star*), which has been cut and sutured back to increase the exposure.

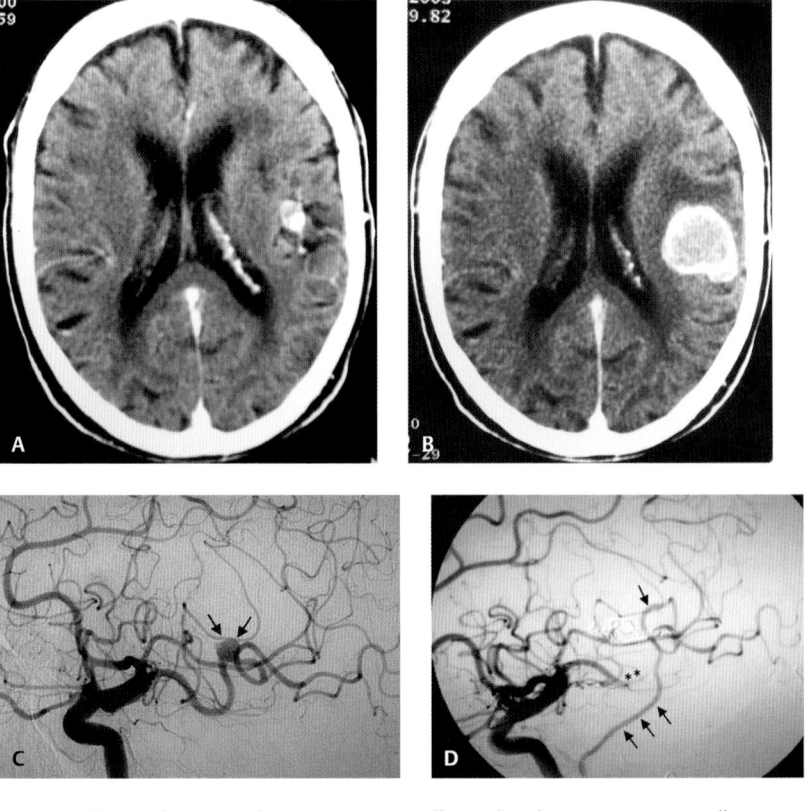

Fig. 9.9 **(A)** Axial CT scan demonstrates a small peripheral MCA aneurysm. Follow-up with serial imaging was recommended. **(B)** Follow-up scan 3 years later reveals dramatic enlargement of the aneurysm with development of associated cerebral edema. **(C)** Lateral digital subtraction angiographic image demonstrates the filling portion of the irregular, fusiform lesion (*arrows*). Of note is the unusually large caliber of the parent artery given its peripheral location. **(D)** Lateral intraoperative common carotid angiographic image demonstrates trapping of the aneurysm with clips. The STA (*3 arrows*) has been anastomosed (*single arrow*) to the parent artery immediately distal to the clips and now irrigates the sacrificed parent artery. The parent artery demonstrates minimal retrograde thrombosis (*asterisks*). The aneurysm was opened and evacuated of thrombus, resulting in immediate postoperative improvement in the patient's severe, progressive speech difficulty. The treatment of the lesion is seen in 🔘 VIDEO 50 . (*Images reprinted with permission from the Journal of Neurosurgery.*)

Truly fusiform aneurysms are uncommon, but they do occur, and many result from dissections 🔘 VIDEO 52 (**Fig. 9.10**). They can be located anywhere along the course of an intracranial artery. Some arteries can be sacrificed safely either endovascularly or with an open approach; others cannot. Options for treating truly fusiform aneurysms include circumferential wrapping, clip reconstruction, or trapping

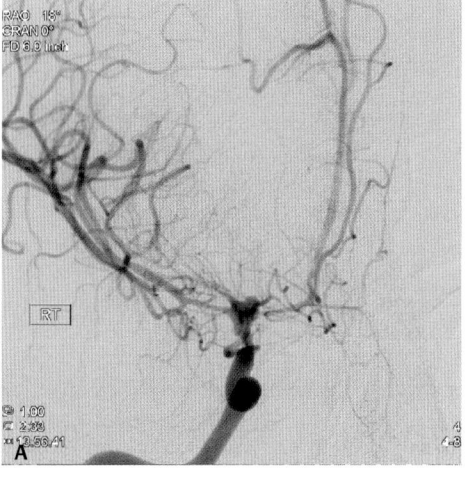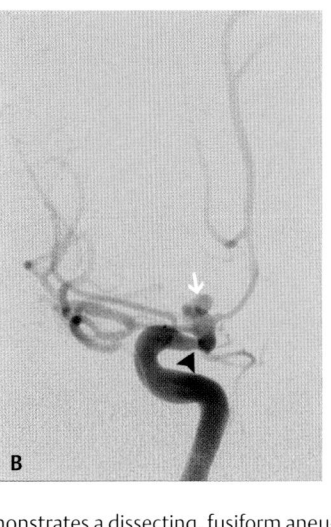

Fig. 9.10 **(A)** AP right internal carotid arteriogram demonstrates a dissecting, fusiform aneurysm of the supraclinoid ICA in a young man who presents with an SAH and right hemispheric ischemia. **(B)** Corresponding lateral arteriographic image reveals local narrowing and irregularity (*black arrowhead*) of the proximal supraclinoid ICA with aneurysmal change (*white arrow*) more distally. The lesion was treated using STA-MCA bypass and sacrifice of the supraclinoid ICA. The treatment of this lesion is shown in ▶ VIDEO 52 .

with or without distal revascularization. There may well be perforators arising from the fusiform segment, and the consequences of sacrificing these vessels must be considered as part of any surgical plan. For example, to avoid a brainstem ischemic event, we do not trap proximal posterior inferior cerebellar artery (PICA) dissections with brainstem perforators arising from the affected segment. Similarly, we would not intentionally sacrifice M1 perforating vessels as part of a trapping procedure, to avoid a capsular injury.

In our experience, gauze or Gore-Tex can be wrapped circumferentially around many of these lesions, snugged tightly, and then secured in place with a clip. If needed, several pieces of material can be used or slits can be created to allow room for small perforators to exit. Several videos demonstrating the treatment of fusiform aneurysms have been included in this series.

■ Previously Coiled Aneurysms

Aneurysms filled with coils represent a unique and challenging subset of lesions for microsurgeons. Because of the explosion of enthusiasm for endovascular treatment of aneurysms over the past two decades, we are encountering an increasing number of aneurysms that have been previously coiled and have recurred. Although many can be treated with repeated coiling, some are failing repeatedly, probably because of a hemodynamic stress that is causing continued pressure on the coil mass, resulting in either direct coil compaction or persisting enlargement of the aneurysm itself. This has created a true challenge for surgeons who are faced with the open microsurgical treatment of aneurysms that are no longer soft and compliant but are full of platinum wire. We have, at times, opened previously coiled aneurysms to remove the coils and enable clip placement (**Fig. 9.11**). With the growing use of coated coils that encourage local scarring, we have found an increased incidence of coils that are intimately adherent to the thin aneurysm wall, and this has made coil removal all but impossible without potentially ripping the aneurysm wall at its neck in some cases.

Some previously coiled aneurysms can be clipped below the existing coil mass (**Figs. 9.12–9.15**). Although it may appear that there is sufficient room below a coil mass to place a clip, we have in many cases found the three-dimensional anatomy to be such that these recurrent or residual necks cannot be clipped without compromising the parent artery (**Fig. 9.16**). Therefore, we have used a distal revascularization procedure with parent artery occlusion in many of these cases. Several videos showing clipping of previously coiled aneurysms have been included in this series ⏵ VIDEO 53 ⏵ VIDEO 54 ⏵ VIDEO 55 (**Fig. 9.17**). The complexity associated with these operations should not be underestimated.

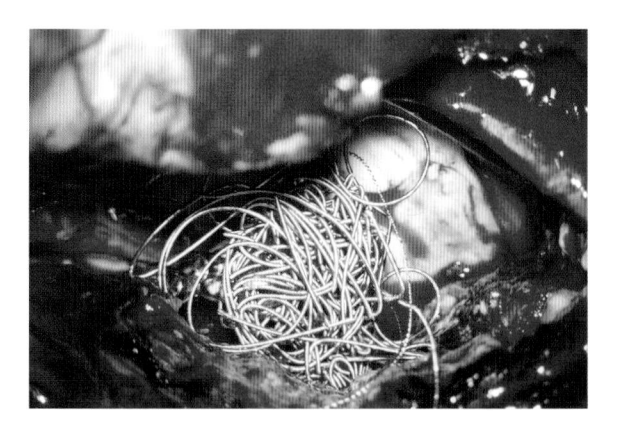

Fig. 9.11 A large coil mass has been removed from a ruptured PCommA aneurysm in preparation for proper neck clipping.

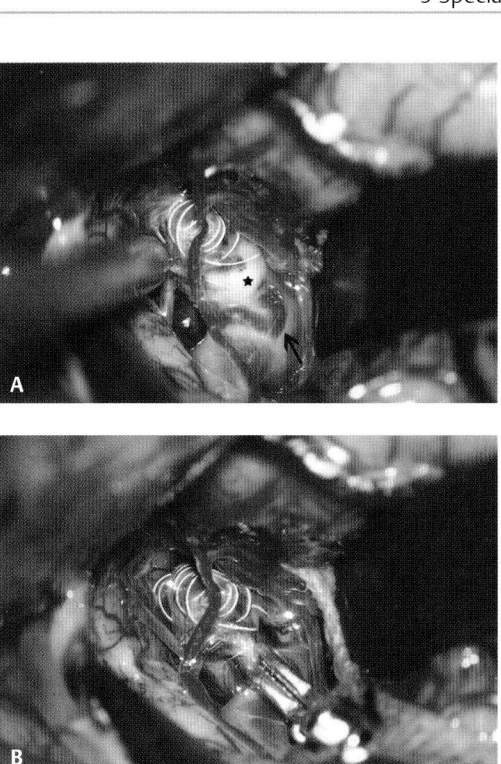

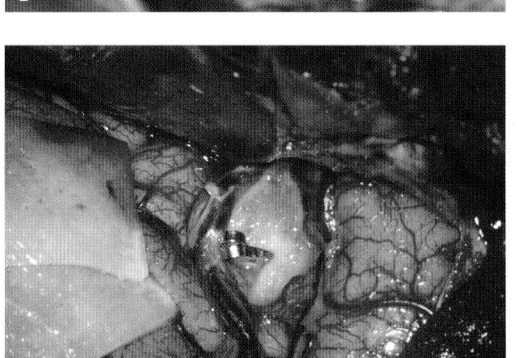

Fig. 9.12 **(A)** A previously coiled MCA aneurysm has been exposed by opening the Sylvian fissure. Note the thinned-out area at the aneurysm neck (*arrow*), the area of open aneurysm (*star*), and the coils readily visible through the aneurysm wall. **(B)** The aneurysm has been repaired with a clip below the coils. **(C)** The extent of the Sylvian opening is shown.

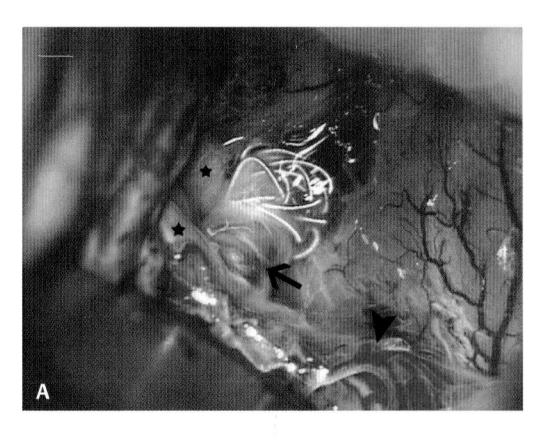

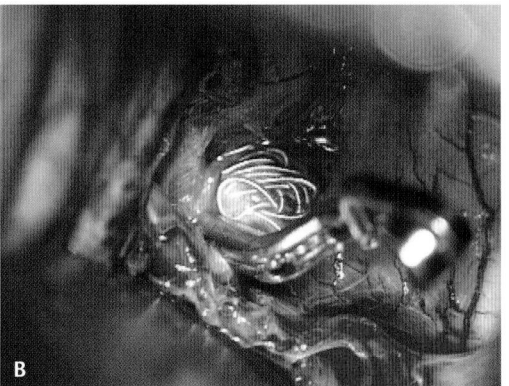

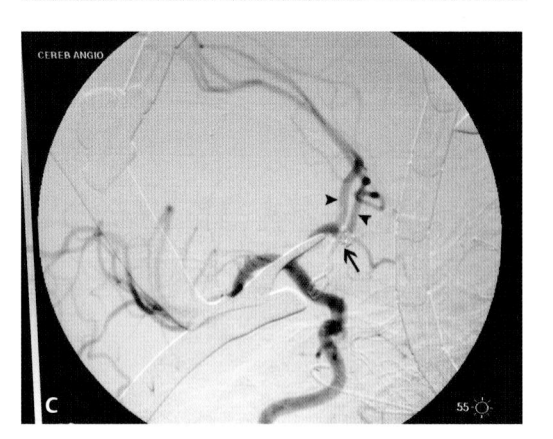

Fig. 9.13 **(A)** A previously coiled ACommA aneurysm has been exposed above the optic nerves. The recurrent thin-walled aneurysm (*arrow*), the A1 segment (*arrowhead*), and both A2 vessels (*stars*) are visible. **(B)** A clip has been applied below the coil mass. **(C)** Intraoperative angiography demonstrates occlusion of the aneurysm (*arrow*) with normal filling of both A2 vessels (*arrowheads*).

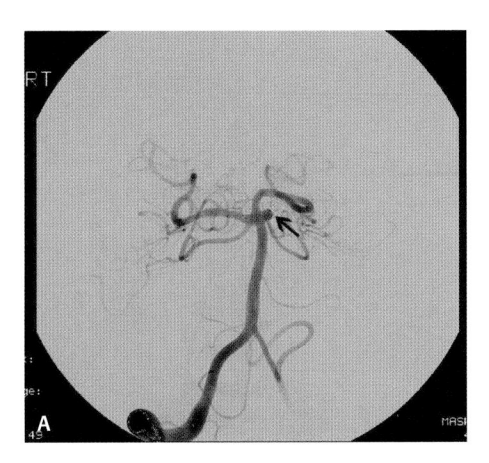

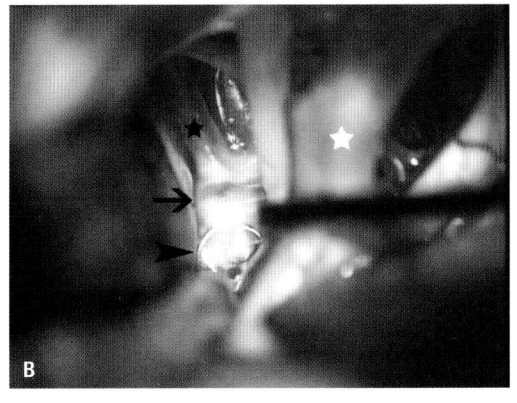

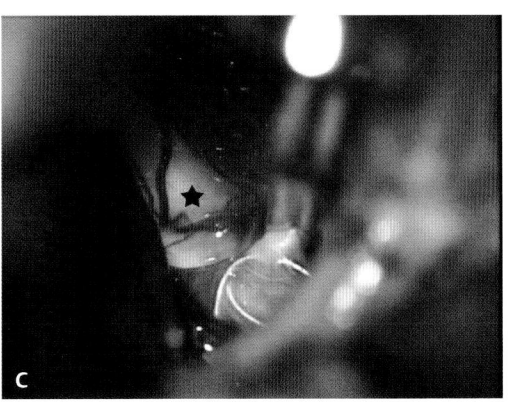

Fig. 9.14 **(A)** A recurrent aneurysm (*arrow*) involving the left superior cerebellar artery origin is shown in this anteroposterior vertebral arteriogram in a patient who had originally present-ed with a severe SAH. **(B)** The aneurysm is exposed through a left pterional craniotomy. The coil mass (*arrowhead*), recurrent aneurysm (*arrow*), and superior cerebellar artery (*black star*) are all seen. The ICA (*white star*) is retracted forward along with the third nerve, using a dissec-tor, to reveal the pertinent anatomy. **(C)** The aneurysm has been clipped. The white brainstem (*star*) is visible in the background. *(Continued on page 116)*

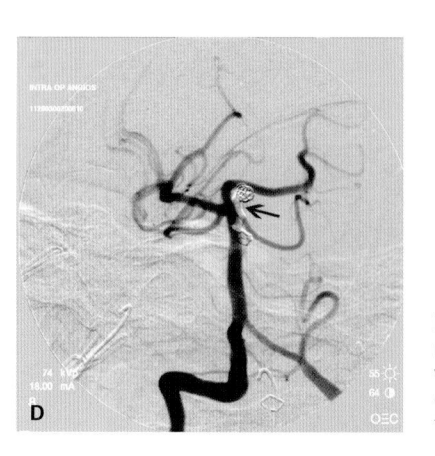

Fig. 9.14 *(Continued)* **(D)** Proper clip placement to obliterate the aneurysm *(arrow)* without compromising flow into the superior cerebellar artery is confirmed with intraoperative angiography.

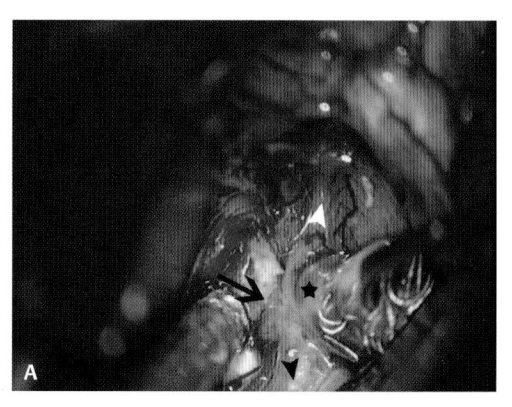

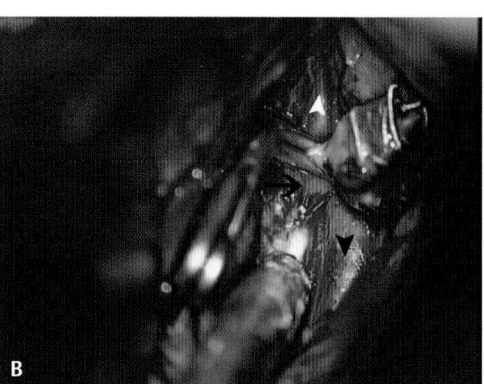

Fig. 9.15 **(A)** A recurrent distal ACA aneurysm has been exposed through an interhemispheric approach to reveal the proximal ACA *(arrow)*, the recurrent aneurysm neck *(star)*, the pericallosal artery *(black arrowhead)*, and the callosomarginal artery *(white arrowhead)*. **(B)** The aneurysm has been clipped. The vessels are again labeled.

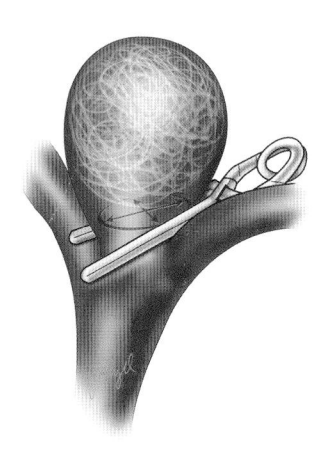

Fig. 9.16 Artist's illustration of a previously coiled aneurysm. The three-dimensional geometry of the coil mass interferes with proper clip closure below the coils, forcing the clip to slip down toward the parent artery.

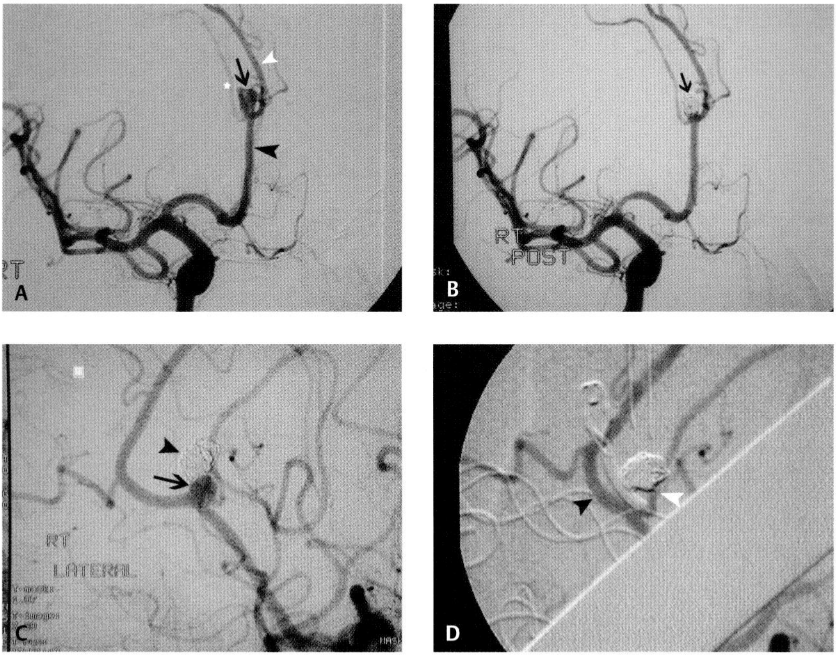

Fig. 9.17 **(A)** A ruptured pericallosal aneurysm (*black arrow*) is shown on a right internal carotid arteriogram along with the proximal ACA (*black arrowhead*), the pericallosal artery (*star*), and the larger callosomarginal vessel (*white arrowhead*). **(B)** The aneurysm was coiled (*arrow*) with a good initial appearance. **(C)** One-year follow-up revealed recurrence of the aneurysm (*arrow*) below the coil mass (*arrowhead*). **(D)** The lesion was clipped below the coil mass, with intraoperative angiography revealing normal filling of the pericallosal (*white arrowhead*) and callosomarginal (*black arrowhead*) arteries. This lesion is treated in ⟳ VIDEO 55 .

■ Rare Locations

Technically, aneurysms can occur anywhere brain arteries are found. The vast majority occur on the proximal vessels of the circle of Willis. When treating aneurysms in unusual locations, one should apply the same basic principles of aneurysm surgery used to treat lesions in the more common sites along the circle of Willis. The same techniques of sharp microsurgical dissection, identifying the relevant anatomy, achieving early proximal control, and obliterating the aneurysm can be used. Challenges may include reaching the aneurysm through an unfamiliar approach and finding a lesion that may be hidden deeply within a fissure.

Many of these aneurysms will be located on peripheral arterial branches. In our experience, a high percentage of these lesions are fusiform, and we have used bypass techniques liberally to treat these lesions. We have favored open surgical exploration in these cases, as opposed to endovascular parent artery occlusion. In fact, many of these lesions can be primarily reconstructed with clips (**Fig. 9.18**). Otherwise, to avoid an ischemic injury, some attempt at distal revascularization has always been appealing from an intuitive perspective.

In this section we have included a video of a rare ruptured lenticulostriate aneurysm in a patient with moyamoya disease ⏩ VIDEO 56 (**Fig. 9.19**) and an unusual spinal aneurysm that had ruptured, producing a severe SAH ⏩ VIDEO 57 (**Fig. 9.20**).

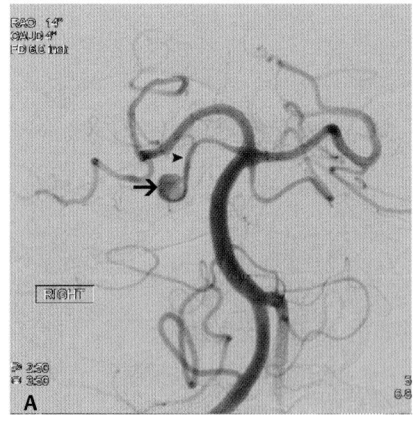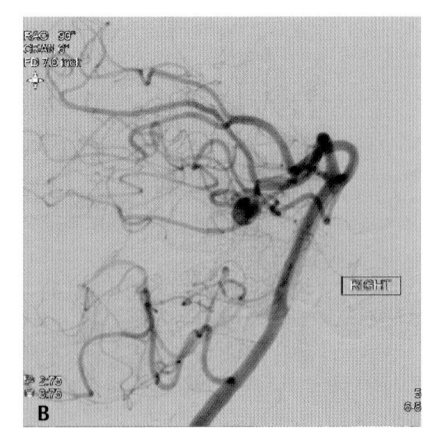

Fig. 9.18 **(A)** Anteroposterior vertebral arteriogram demonstrates a fusiform aneurysm (*arrow*) involving the right SCA (*arrowhead*). **(B)** Corresponding lateral arteriographic image.

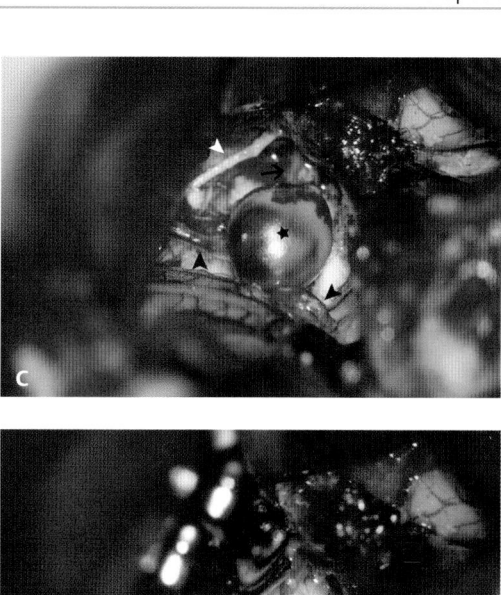

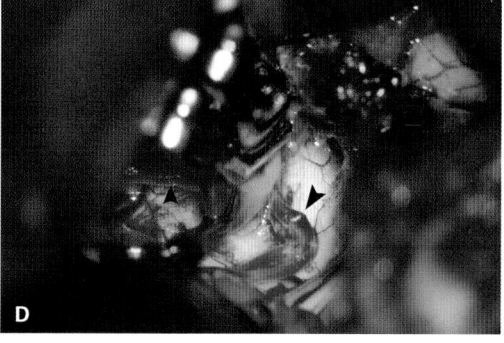

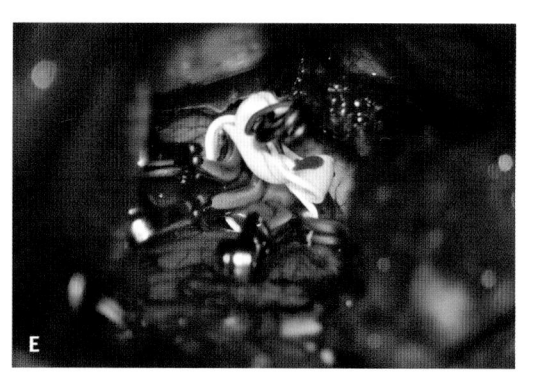

Fig. 9.18 *(Continued)*   **(C)** A peripheral fusiform aneurysm (*star*) of the SCA is exposed through a combined subtemporal-presigmoid approach. The SCA is seen both proximal (*arrow*) and then distal (*black arrowheads*) to the aneurysm, with two separate branches of the artery emerging from the aneurysm. The fourth cranial nerve (*white arrowhead*) is seen crossing the field. **(D)** The aneurysm has been reconstructed with multiple clips, and the two efferent SCA branches are seen (*arrowheads*). **(E)** Gore-Tex has been wrapped around the clip construct.

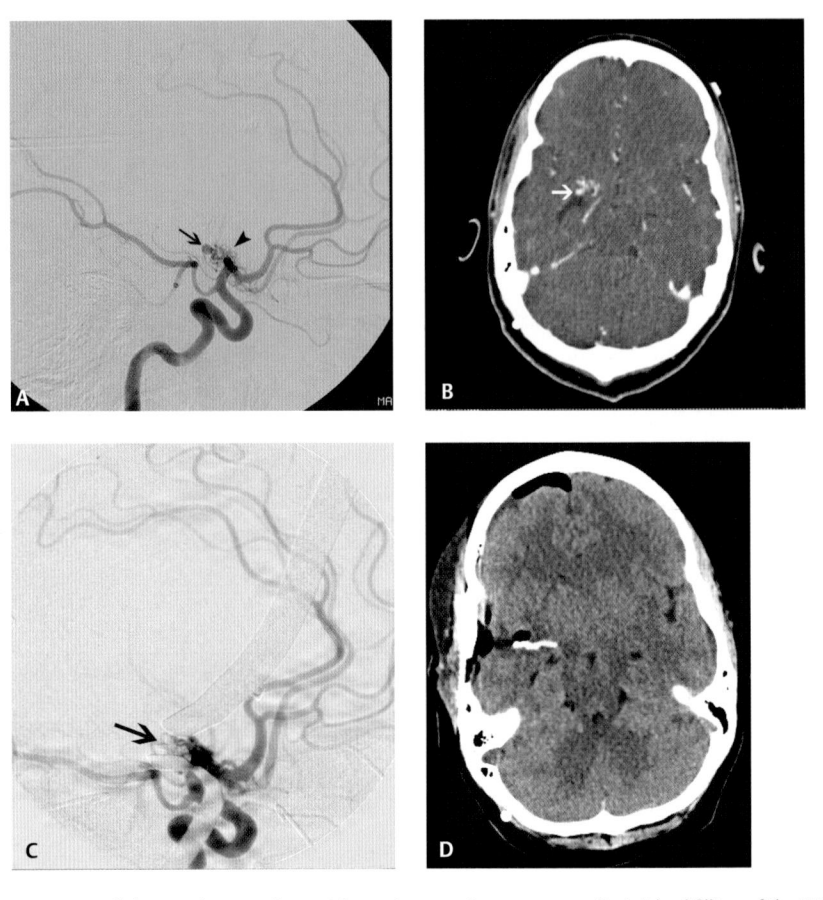

Fig. 9.19 **(A)** Lateral internal carotid arteriogram demonstrates diminished filling of the MCA territory associated with moyamoya changes (*arrowhead*) with a posteriorly directed lenticulostriate aneurysm (*arrow*) that had bled previously, resulting in a temporal lobe hematoma with intraventricular extension. The patient underwent an unsuccessful attempted EC-IC bypass at another facility. A decision was made to clip the aneurysm and then redo the bypass. **(B)** Axial CT image with intravenous contrast reveals the aneurysm (*arrow*). **(C)** Intraoperative lateral angiographic image demonstrates clip occlusion of the aneurysm (*arrow*). **(D)** Postoperative axial CT scan reveals the transtemporal trajectory and the final location of the clip. The treatment of this lesion is shown in ⚙ VIDEO 56).

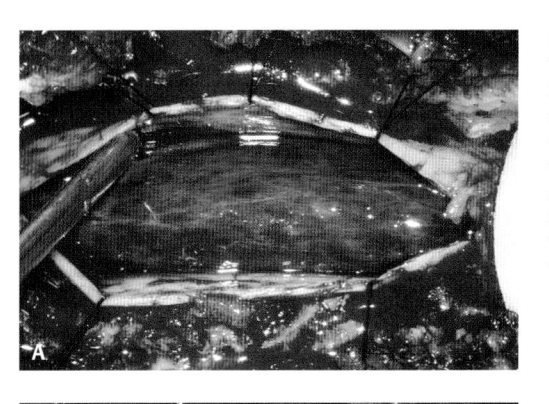

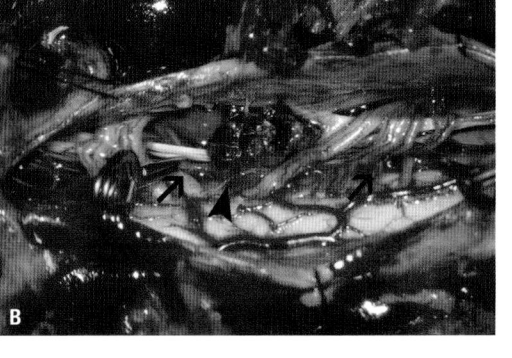

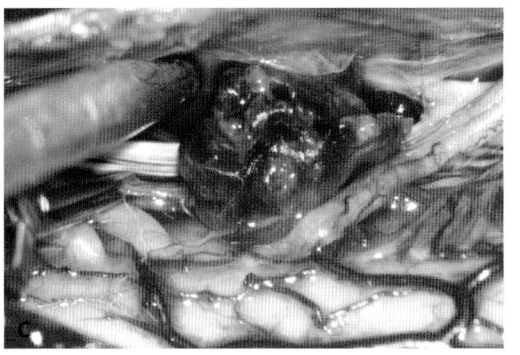

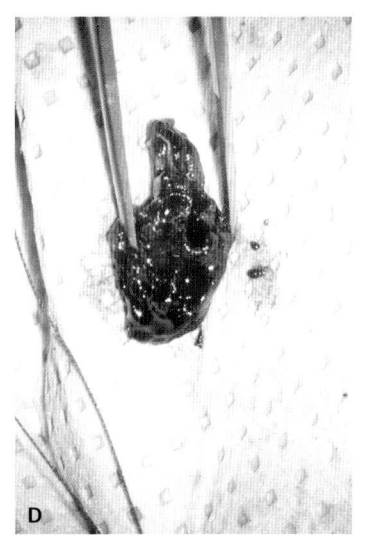

Fig. 9.20 **(A)** A cervical laminoplasty has been performed to expose the SAH visible immediately upon dural opening. **(B)** The ruptured aneurysm (*arrowhead*) and the small vessel upon which it arose (*arrows*) are seen. **(C)** A magnified view of the aneurysm is shown. **(D)** The aneurysm has been trapped and excised. This lesion is treated in VIDEO 57.

■ Aneurysms Associated with AVMs

Aneurysms associated with arteriovenous malformations (AVMs) represent a unique subgroup of lesions that are generally flow-related. They will often regress if the AVM is treated, but they may also represent the source of bleeding that brings an AVM to light. In general, we have used endovascular options to treat ruptured feeding artery aneurysms when possible.

10 General Principles of Aneurysm Surgery: Nuances and Advice for Successful Outcomes and Complication Avoidance

There are some general principles that can be applied to any microsurgical procedure for the treatment of intracranial aneurysms. These are points that have been important in achieving a successful outcome in the vast majority of cases in the author's personal experience. It should be noted that there is rarely "one right way" to do anything in neurosurgery. What works well for one surgeon may not be appropriate for another. Nevertheless, these are some general rules that have been particularly useful to the author.

■ Patient Selection

The surgeon's struggle to achieve reliably excellent results in the treatment of intracranial aneurysms begins not in the operating room but with judicious patient selection. Treatment should be recommended for unruptured aneurysms only if the surgeon is confident that the surgery can be performed safely, given the relatively benign natural history associated with simple observation. In the setting of a ruptured lesion, the improved durability associated with surgical clipping as opposed to endovascular therapy becomes meaningless if surgery results in a poor immediate neurological outcome from which the patient never recovers. In many ways, patient selection represents at least "half the battle."

■ There Is No Substitute for an Organized Plan

Although aneurysm surgery demands a certain amount of flexibility based on intraoperative findings, a good aneurysm surgeon will have an organized plan of attack, including potential contingency options should things change during surgery.

■ Expose What You Must, No More and No Less

Obviously, it is impossible to expose precisely and only the absolutely necessary anatomy in every operation. Nevertheless, a good neurovascular surgeon will over time develop a sense for just how much exposure is needed to complete the task at hand. This does not mean that one never increases the exposure by further opening a fissure, for example. But there is no need to open the Sylvian fissure widely to reach every anterior circulation aneurysm, and the author has seen surgeons get into trouble exposing, for example, the middle cerebral arterial branches unnecessarily to treat a carotid ophthalmic aneurysm.

▧ Achieve Your Primary Objective First

When treating multiple aneurysms, there is usually a larger, more concerning, or even ruptured lesion as well as a smaller or asymptomatic aneurysm of lesser concern. At times, the smaller lesion must be dealt with en route to the real target. Nevertheless, one should generally avoid the temptation to treat the smaller or less concerning aneurysm first. The author has seen surgeons get into trouble with a small asymptomatic middle cerebral artery (MCA) bifurcation aneurysm, forcing them to end an operation before ever reaching the main target, such as a large anterior communicating lesion.

▧ Use Sharp Dissection

As a general rule, sharp dissection is safer than blunt "tearing." At the same time, we will often use gentle blunt dissection to break fine arachnoid bands during the opening of the fissure, and we have illustrated this repeatedly in the videos in this series. But once you're working down near the aneurysm, sharp dissection with a knife or microscissors is preferred.

▧ Don't Force It

It's important for an aneurysm surgeon to develop a sense of what he or she can and cannot do. These are delicate structures, and blunt force rarely works well. By maximizing dissection of the aneurysm and its surrounding structures, I often find that the clipping is rather anti-climactic. All the anatomy has already been exposed. A clip has been tested for the proper shape and size, and simply applying the clip and letting it close should be quick and easy.

▧ Common Sense Always Rules

If it doesn't look right, if it doesn't feel safe, then you need to think twice. When it looks as though I haven't adequately prepared for a situation in which I find myself, I will often tell myself, "Take a step back, and think about this . . ."

The neurosurgeon should always remember that there is nothing wrong with exploring an aneurysm and deciding it is too complicated to treat safely with primary clip occlusion. Although some aneurysms are better suited for open microsurgery, that fact does not absolutely preclude the possibility of an endovascular approach, at times with a stent if the parent arteries are of adequate caliber. Therefore, if a surgeon is in the operating room and cannot adequately identify the critical anatomy necessary for precise clip placement, it may be quite reasonable to stop and refer the patient for an attempt at endovascular treatment or to a more experienced microsurgeon if endovascular therapy is not considered feasible. In fact, this is generally a much better approach than to "force" the situation and potentially end up with a severe neurological injury. On many occasions, even when our endovascular colleagues had previously recommended open microsurgical treatment, we have called them to the operating room for an intraoperative consultation to discuss the potential for an endovascular approach when we have unexpectedly encountered a situation that is felt to increase significantly the risk of proceeding with direct clip reconstruction. In general, patients are warned preoperatively that there is a remote possibility that we will not primarily clip the aneurysm if the intraoperative findings alter our assessment of the "risk/benefit" profile associated with proceeding.

■ Avoid "Point of No Return" Situations Whenever Possible

At times, there is no good choice other than to cross a line of "no return." A good example might be opening an aneurysm to perform an aneurysmorrhaphy for clip reconstruction. Of course, once that aneurysm is cut open, there is always the possibility that you will not be able to reconstruct the vessel with clips. I have avoided these situations whenever possible. For example, prior to attempting aneurysmorrhaphy, I prefer to do a distal bypass. Then there is no "time limit" to the temporary arterial occlusion, and if you can't reconstruct the aneurysm, the segment can be left trapped.

■ Rehearse Mentally

Rehearsing an upcoming surgery in your mind is a good way to prepare. There are some simple tricks that can make this easier. When reviewing the imaging studies, orienting the pictures, particularly the angiograms, in the way you will encounter the anatomy at the time of surgery can help you visualize the important structures. When using three-dimensional rotational angiography, the surgeon can use the image-processing machine to view the relevant vascular anatomy from a variety of perspectives, helping to visualize those structures that will be encountered and those that will be hidden during the surgical exposure. In addition, thinking about the steps of the surgery, including what you would do if things don't go as planned, can help prepare you for potential intraoperative issues.

■ Temporary Clips Are Great When Needed

Many aneurysm surgeons use temporary clips on every case. I do not. It's a matter of personal preference. I find that too many temporary clips can hinder the exposure, potentially damage fine perforators, and prevent proper permanent clip application. That said, temporary clips are critical in some settings, such as basilar apex aneurysms of any meaningful size and when dealing with a difficult ruptured aneurysm.

■ Consider Adenosine

Adenosine is a great drug. About ten years ago, I was operating on a patient with a ruptured somewhat fusiform anterior communicating artery (ACommA) aneurysm on a feeding artery to a high-flow arteriovenous malformation (AVM). The aneurysm ruptured, and I simply could not adequately visualize the structures to achieve proper control. We infused adenosine, transiently stopped the heart, and clipped the aneurysm. We reported this in the literature, and we have subsequently heard from numerous surgeons who have used this technique to salvage what could have been an intraoperative catastrophe.

■ Use Retractors Properly

There is no question that over-retraction can result in brain injury. Given this, there has been a growing trend moving away from the use of brain retractors in all forms of neurosurgery. Over time, I have decreased the use of retractors during surgery, but I still believe there is an important role for the use of brain retractors in aneurysm surgery. Instead of using the retractors to *move* and *hold* the brain out of the way, we use retractors to *protect* the brain from inadvertent injury while working past structures that are out of focus through the operating microscope. In general, I feel comfortable with the use of retractors when I can remove the retractor and the brain remains essentially in the same position anyway. Of note, I have always been concerned that when treating a ruptured aneurysm, if the aneurysm were to rebleed without retractors in place, the bleeding could become problematic. Most of the videos in this series include the use of soft, malleable, Teflon-coated brain retractors.

■ Don't Sacrifice Arteries or Veins Unless You Must

One should sacrifice vessels as infrequently as possible. With that said, occasionally, a Sylvian vein will be placed under great tension to expose a tough, ruptured aneurysm. In such a case, if the aneurysm were to rebleed intraoperatively, the vein would likely be torn during attempts to control the aneurysm, potentially making the situation even worse. The surgeon must carefully weigh the risks and benefits of each maneuver in cases such as this. At times, it may be worthwhile to sacrifice a small vein to facilitate a successful procedure.

Longer Is Not Better

At some point, it seems that people began to believe that a long operation is somehow indicative of a "well-fought" battle. The implication is that surgery for the treatment of an intracranial aneurysm should take many hours (four, six, even eight hours), if it is to be done well. With a methodical and organized approach, most aneurysms can be treated in less than two hours from beginning to end of surgery. Although particularly difficult aneurysms may require more time, simple anterior circulation and upper basilar aneurysms generally do not, and a longer surgery puts the brain at risk for secondary injury. Ultimately, take the time you need, but shorter is better in my experience.

If You Make a Mistake, Relax and Try to Fix It

Every surgeon, no matter how experienced, makes mistakes. Sometimes they are minor, but occasionally they are more serious. The good aneurysm surgeon must train him- or herself to stay calm when this happens, as it will inevitably. Can the situation be repaired? If not, what are some options? For example, I can recall one case when dissection at the neck of an ACommA aneurysm resulted in a small tear. Temporary clips were applied to stop the bleeding, but it was clear that the only way to stop the bleeding permanently would be to bring a clip across the origin of one of the A2 vessels. Instead, we were able to place two strategic 10–0 sutures at the level of the tear, allowing us to keep the clip above the A2 origin. This could never have been done without maintaining a calm demeanor and taking the time to assess all options carefully. If unsuccessful, I would have considered an intraoperative angiogram to assess collateral to the distal anterior cerebral artery (ACA) territory involved, and a distal bypass might have been an option.

Your Endovascular Colleagues Are Your Best Friends, Not Your Enemies

Too many neurosurgeons still think interventional neuroradiologists or surgeons who coil aneurysms are the enemy. This is not a competition. By collaborating on every case, you will be able to optimize outcomes for your patients, limit your own surgical misadventures, and become a far better aneurysm surgeon.

◼ Ask For Help When You're Not Sure

After completing residency or fellowship training, many neurosurgeons begin their practice and assume that they are or should be "on their own." Being unsure and asking for help after so many years of training can be thought of as a sign of weakness and even incompetence. In fact, asking for another opinion is often a sign of maturity and self-confidence. If a young vascular neurosurgeon enters a practice with a more senior neurovascular colleague, it will be easy to discuss complex cases. But if the young surgeon takes a position at an academic center or private hospital where he or she is the only vascular neurosurgeon, it can be more difficult to ask for help when it's needed. At the start of my career, I frequently sought the opinion of expert neurovascular surgeons, including Dr. Charles Drake, and others with whom I had spent time during my training. Today, I still ask for opinions on complex cases when I'm unsure how best to proceed. The ability to ask for help when uncertain is an important tool that is often underutilized by neurosurgeons, who tend to be highly independent by nature.

On a similar note, it is important for younger neurosurgeons to recognize and remember that learning doesn't end at the conclusion of residency or fellowship. In many ways, this is really the beginning! Working with a more experienced colleague early in his or her career can be extremely beneficial to the young neurovascular surgeon and even more beneficial to his or her patients. In an era when open microsurgery should be performed only when outcomes are clearly better than those offered by endovascular options (or the natural history of the underlying condition), younger surgeons should seek opportunities to work collaboratively with more experienced neurovascular surgeons during the early stages of their careers.

◼ Do the Right Thing . . . You Won't Regret It!

Neurosurgery is a funny profession. There is no escaping the fact that ego can become your enemy. I recall a particular case in which an angiogram of a complex basilar apex aneurysm was sent to me, and I was immediately enthusiastic about the potential for a challenging open surgical procedure. Then, when the patient actually came to visit me in the office . . . with her husband and three young children . . . reality set in. I knew that I could offer the patient a reasonable chance for a favorable outcome, but I also knew that this particular aneurysm would be more safely treated with endovascular coiling. In this situation (and many others like it), I had to decide which was more important: satisfying my ego by recommending surgery or doing what I believed was right by sending the patient for endovascular therapy.

I have always tried to do what I know in my heart is right, and I have never regretted it for more than a fleeting moment. At times, after considering all the options, the patient requests the open surgery anyway. But even when the patient does not,

I am convinced that you cannot be a great surgeon if you are making recommendations based on what you want to do rather than based upon what the patient needs.

By the same token, no one starts their career as a great aneurysm surgeon. Over time, it is hoped that one improves, but along the way, the neurovascular surgeon will encounter complex cases that may be better treated by a more experienced surgeon. In my practice, whenever I have felt there would be a "measurable" difference in terms of the likelihood for a good outcome for a particular patient, I have offered to refer that patient to a more experienced surgeon. Over the years, I have sent many patients across the country to obtain what I believe represented a better chance at an excellent result. Again, I have never regretted these decisions. Although there may be benefits in terms of more rapidly gaining expertise associated with keeping and personally operating on all these cases, when one remembers these are people and not just medical record numbers or opportunities for a great surgery, the right decision comes into focus.

Index

Note: Page numbers followed by *f* and *t* indicate figures and tables, respectively.